CONTEMPORARY ISSUES IN Nursing 1

To Matthew Jack

For Churchill Livingstone:

Commisioning editors: Peter Shepherd, Alex Mathieson
Project development editor: Valerie Bain
Project manager: Valerie Burgess
Project controller: Derek Robertson
Copy editor: Holly Regan-Jones
Design direction: Judith Wright
Sales promotion executive: Hilary Brown

CONTEMPORARY ISSUES IN Nursing 1

Edited by

Francis C. Biley
Lecturer in Nursing, University of Wales College of Medicine,
School of Nursing Studies, Cardiff, UK

Christopher Maggs
RCN Professor of Nursing Research, University of Wales College of Medicine,
School of Nursing Studies, Cardiff, UK

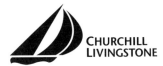

**CHURCHILL
LIVINGSTONE**

NEW YORK, EDINBURGH, LONDON, MADRID, MELBOURNE, SAN FRANCISCO, TOKYO 1996

CHURCHILL LIVINGSTONE
Medical Division of Pearson Professional Limited

Distributed in the United States of America by Churchill
Livingstone, 650 Avenue of the Americas, New York, N.Y. 10011,
and by associated companies, branches and representatives
throughout the world.

First published 1996

ISBN 0 443 053510

British Library Cataloguing in Publication Data
A catalogue record for this book is available from the British Library.

Library of Congress Cataloging in Publication Data
A catalog record for this book is available from the Library of Congress.

The
publisher's
policy is to use
**paper manufactured
from sustainable forests**

Produced through Longman Malaysia, PP

Contents

Introduction   vi

Contributors   xi

SECTION 1   Research   **1**

1. Laughing at death: the ultimate paradox
   Catriona Knight   3

2. Skin-to-skin contact for premature and sick infants and
   their mothers
   Kim Smith   31

3. The readability of patient information
   Duncan Goodes   79

4. Patients' and nurses' experiences of feeding: a phenomenological
   study
   Jan Dewing   113

SECTION 2   Reviews   **171**

5. Primary nursing: a feminist perspective
   Rayna McDonald-Birch   173

6. Spirituality in nursing: towards an unfolding of the mystery
   Louise S. Morgan   203

7. The most significant 'nothing': a concept analysis of
   personal space
   Karen Poole   233

Introduction

This collection of student dissertations in nursing and midwifery science is a celebration. First, the volume celebrates the academic work of some recent students of nursing and midwifery, either as they prepare for initial or post-registration practice or as they develop a deeper understanding of the profession of which they have been a part for, perhaps, many years. Second, it celebrates the nature of the contribution that scholarship makes to professional development. Third, it demonstrates the considerable professional pride that we, as teachers and facilitators of professional and personal development, have in our students.

The volume is also something of a first. It provides a unique opportunity for a wider dissemination of the academic work of students of nursing and midwifery. Too often, student dissertations in their entirety are read by examiners and then relegated to the shelf. In addition to the message this may give to students about the value of their work, it seems a regrettable waste of intellectual (and emotional) energy on the part of all involved.

The contributions presented here are largely in their original versions; that is, as presented for examination. Most examination regulations state that dissertations are expected to be a 'significant piece of work' by the student and are usually at least 10 000 or 20 000 words long. They are often considered too long for conventional magazine or journal publication. At the same time, such a length would normally be considered to be too short or inappropriate for publication as a small book, monograph or even as an occasional paper. We believe that this publication is the first to provide a vehicle or opportunity for students of nursing and midwifery to publish their works in their entirety, without the need to pad out the content in order to create an individual work of book length, or reduce the length of their work by perhaps 30, 50 or even 75% in order for it to be of suitable length for journal publication. How much of the essence of a study is lost during this process? This collection permits longer dissertation studies to reach a wider audience and therefore to have the opportunity to have a much greater impact on the future of nursing and midwifery practice than if they had just been forgotten and left to languish on some dusty shelf in a nursing or midwifery library.

There is also an element of the lesson plan here. So often, students will ask us, as teachers, facilitators or as supervisors of study, to define the exact nature of the dissertation, whether at undergraduate or postgraduate level, and we discuss issues such as analysis, synthesis and thesis, reviewing literature, presentation of ideas and data, formulating research proposals and more. We may send the student off to the library to read what others have written and to see how they constructed their dissertations, and we hold seminars to discuss the practicalities of summative dissertations and research. The contributions in this volume are all by recent Bachelor and Masters degree graduates of various institutes of higher and further education from around the United Kingdom. They are, then, one highly visible answer to the perennial question – what is a dissertation? Read this volume to find out not only about a series of fascinating subjects and research studies, many of which should be considered central to the practice of high quality, contemporary nursing and midwifery practice, but also to find out how dissertations are constructed; how that last, vital stage of study is completed.

Finally, the collection is about accountability. Each of the dissertations presented here has been discussed and agreed between teacher and student, supervised and monitored, marked by internal and external examiners and each passed, with varying degrees of success, and has therefore been regarded as meeting, in part, the requirements for the relevant award. We are thus 'opening our books' to a wider audience who will then be in a position to judge whether we, as teachers or facilitators and students, meet the standards and expectations of others.

We do so with neither diffidence nor arrogance. There are only a few occasions when we can, in all honesty, say that what we have read is the definitive statement on a given subject. The nature of knowledge and the construction of professional knowledge in particular are in flux. The authors of these dissertations, therefore, do not present their studies as final in any sense but as contributions to that process of change. In so doing, they are also exposing their work to a wider (and perhaps more critical?) audience of their peers.

We have great pleasure in including the seven chapters in this volume. As we have already stated, the content of each chapter was initially developed and presented as a course-work dissertation in part fulfilment of an undergraduate or postgraduate degree in nursing or midwifery. There were no explicit criteria for inclusion of these dissertations in this volume, but readers will agree that all of the subjects chosen show a high degree of innovation and imagination, are creative in the way that they handle their subjects and, of course, the subjects are central to the practice of high quality, contemporary nursing and midwifery. This is typified by the excellent contributions from Jan Dewing, a lecturer/practitioner and senior nurse at the reknowned Burford Nursing Development Unit in Oxfordshire, who explored the experiences of being fed and of feeding from a phenomenological perspective (one of the first, if not the first, study of its kind), and from Karen Poole, who explored a critically important concept, that of personal space, again an area that has had little emphasis placed on it in the nursing literature.

The quality to be found in undergraduate and postgraduate dissertations is further reflected in the other chapters. Rayna McDonald-Birch, who is currently a PhD student studying nursing care of the elderly throughout Europe, explores primary nursing from an entirely new, feminist, perspective; Louise Morgan contributes very usefully to the debate on spirituality, highlighting its considerable significance for everyday nursing practice; and Duncan Goodes explores the readability of patient information literature in his chapter of that name.

Finally, the use of 'black' or thanatological humour by nurses working in palliative care is sensitively explored by Kim Smith, and Catriona Knight makes a very effective contribution to the development of midwifery nursing practice with her chapter studying the effects of 'kangaroo' care on sick infants and their mothers.

It was an enormous pleasure for us to put this collection together. We found all of the chapters stimulating and exciting. Whether you are a student nurse or midwife embarking on your own dissertation project, a nurse or midwife working in a practice setting and wishing in some way to explore new avenues for practice, or an educator keen to explore new developments, we hope that you will enjoy reading this volume as much as we enjoyed constructing it and hope that it will inform you as much as it did us.

1996   FCB and CM

Contributors

Jan Dewing MN BA RGN Dip Nurs Dip Nurs Ed RNT
Lecturer Practitioner, Burford Hospital, Burford

I first became aware that I was not skilled at feeding patients some time after I started working in a unit that provided services for young adults with physical disabilities. Previously I had always assumed that I knew what I was doing, though looking back I cannot remember ever being shown how to feed patients, nor can I recall any other clinical or theoretical teaching experiences that had prepared me for the activity. I realised that I had never considered feeding as a 'real skill.'

I remember talking with a group of patients about the quality of the presentation of meals, after the nurses reported to me that the food trolley was arriving with spilt food. The patients did not seem concerned about this, but in the course of our conversation it became evident that they had views on other issues surrounding mealtimes and the food they were served. They described to me many issues which affected some or all of them. These included the way in which the dining area was arranged, for example, the lack of choice about where they sat and who they had sitting next to them. Some patients mentioned the lack of privacy for eating as it was common for staff to stand around the edges of the dining area.

The dialogue with patients was a key experience for me. I began to observe what was happening at mealtimes, talked again with patients about their experiences and undertook a literature search on the subject. I reflected on the issues involved for some time. I was in a position to change certain aspects of practice but I was unsure if I was changing what patients regarded as priorities for them or whether the new ways would be any more patient centred.

A course at Masters Degree level gave me the opportunity to research the whole experience of feeding in depth and, although it is now some time since I finished my research, I retain an interest in the way people's experiences of feeding are affected by the organization of mealtimes.

Duncan Goodes BNSc FAETC RMN RGN
Surgical Services Manager, Lymington Hospital, Lymington

My current position is that of Surgical Services Manager at Southampton Community Health Services NHS Trust. Previously, I was Charge Nurse on a Men's Medical Ward at Lymington Hospital and a Staff Nurse at Salisbury General Hospital. My Bachelor of Nursing Studies was completed at the Faculty of Medicine, Southampton University. The reasons for choosing to investigate the readability of patient information were many. Working as a Charge Nurse on an acute medical ward at the time the study was commenced I was part of a team caring for patients with a wide variety of presenting conditions. Many of these patients had conditions that would affect their lives on a long-term basis and as such needed information that they could not only discuss with the health care team while in hospital but also utilise after discharge. It was the practice of the ward staff to give written information in support of verbal. Generally we felt we could congratulate ourselves on the care and information patients received but little was done, initially, to critically assess the effectiveness and accessibility to the patient of the written information given.

Two things led to a perceived need to investigate the information we were giving patients: first, I came across an article by Cathy Meade, an American author who had investigated the readability of American patient information booklets and found them wanting and, second, a realisation dawned that patient information booklets that were found useful to learner nurses as part of their learning experience on the ward might not be appropriate to patients. While reading for a Bachelors degree in Nursing Sciences, an opportunity arose to examine a topic of interest in depth. I chose to review literature investigating the readability of patient information. From the literature review performed it became evident that little, if any, research had been conducted on this topic in the UK. North American studies had investigated the readability level of patient literature, not what effect this might have on the patient's perception of the text. Many studies did nothing more than assess the readability of some information and note that it was written at a reading level higher than was thought to be the population average. There was a seemingly very reasonable (albeit often unwritten) assumption made in some of these studies that if difficult text was made easier, this would be better from the patient's perspective. However, the author could find no research that tested this. Hence this short study was undertaken.

Catriona Knight BNSc (Hons) RGN
Staff Nurse, Countess Mountbatten House, Southampton

Having worked in palliative care for 18 months, I had recognized in myself the growing need to develop long-term and short-term coping strategies in order to continue to function effectively within my role.

As a new employee to this environment I had noted and been rather shocked by the subject matter and the use of humour in the palliative care environment. My interest grew to explore why this type of humour was used and what purpose it served within this type of environment.

My exploration started with searching the literature to seek answers to my questions but frustratingly little literature was found on humour, and no literature was found which particularly related to the use of humour by staff in palliative care or other healthcare settings. I therefore decided to seek out some answers for myself, and the idea was born.

This research highlights the need for workers in palliative care to develop a coping strategy in order to function effectively and protect the individual from being emotionally affected by traumatic and painful events.

The study highlights the need for research into coping strategies used in health care in order to utilize them in an attempt to create positive working environments and reduce the risk of 'burnout', often associated with high-stress occupations such as nursing.

It is hoped that this study may alleviate healthcare workers' guilt associated with the use of such humour and to normalize it and justify its use as a valid coping mechanism.

Nurse researchers should develop an awareness that research should not only be predominantly focused on clinical practice but also should examine the environment dynamics that ultimately influence the quality of patient care.

Rayna McDonald-Birch BN (Hons) RGN
Research Nurse, School of Nursing Studies, University of Wales College of Medicine, Cardiff

Since qualifying as a RGN, I have worked as a staff nurse in paediatrics, ITU, ENT and care of the elderly. I completed my Bachelor of Nursing degree at the University of Wales, College of Medicine, and am currently employed there as a research nurse coordinating a multicentre European study.

I chose this topic because, as I started to become familiar with the feminist literature, it seemed to explain many of my personal and professional experiences as a woman and a nurse. I also felt that there were undercurrents of change within the nursing community and that this was a result of 'underground' feminist activity. Primary nursing seemed to embrace a feminist ideology yet this had never been explored in any literature. I felt the common attributes needed to be explicated, labelled as being of feminist orientation and made public. I wanted to portray feminism as a philosophy that would not seem alien to the nurse on the ward and to demystify and demonstrate that the radical feminist stereotype is in reality a product of partriarchal insecurity and vulnerability.

I believe that the consequences for nursing practice resulting from this work are:

- Primary nursing being recognized as a method of organizing care that is based on an ideology that is feminist in orientation.
- Nursing that is demonstrating congruency between theory and practice.
- Nurses challenging the structure and dynamics of the relationships that exist in the healthcare setting, leading towards shared knowledge and power, and a flattening of the hierarchy.
- Primary nursing units creating nursing-centred units, providing the potential for new knowledge to be created inductively.

Louise Morgan BN (Hons) RN (Adult)
Staff Nurse, University Hospital of Wales NHS Trust, Cardiff

Clinical placements during the Bachelor of Nursing course developed my awareness of an area which I believe to be vital to the holistic care of patients, that of spiritual care, an area subject to much misunderstanding and neglect. I had observed many examples of spiritual care, both good and bad, and this led me to examine why nurses seem unable to deal with the spiritual needs of their patients, when they are often in an ideal position to provide such care. The small amount of space allowed for information about religion on our assessment sheets testifies to our lack of interest in anything beyond straightforward labelling.

The dissertation which I submitted for the BN course arose out of a collection of experiences and pertinent incidences, and from an analysis of current literature research and anecdotal evidence. It became clear that there were a number of areas which nurses needed to address:

1. *Lack of self-awareness.* Nurses who do not know their own values and belief systems find difficulty in helping the patient clarify and deal with theirs.

2. *Lack of knowledge about religious, cultural and philosophical beliefs and practices.* Offence caused to patients by ignorance on the part of the nurse does not encourage trust and openness in the nurse-patient relationship. Nurses also tend to avoid religious issues, leaving them to ministers of religion.

3. *Lack of awareness of the spiritual needs of atheists and agnostics.* Atheists have their own belief and value systems but their spiritual needs are often denied by nurses who believe that spirituality and religion are synonymous.

4. *Lack of communication skills and inability to deal with emotions.* If nurses' own feelings, worries and concerns are not encouraged or drawn out then patients may, in turn, feel unable to express *their* emotions.

The aim of my study was to examine the definition and meaning of spirituality as developed by other writers and to explore the research available. Through this I hoped to gain an understanding of spiritual distress and how nurses can intervene in an appropriate and inoffensive way to meet their patients' spiritual needs. The importance of spiritual care for the terminally-ill patient was an area of particular interest to me, but the study was also intended to develop ideas which nurses could adapt and apply to their own workplaces. Ideas for future research also arose from my study.

I took a Judeo-Christian approach for the study, partly because the literature available is set in that context and partly because of my own spirituality. However, all belief systems and ideas have been acknowledged throughout the text and my conclusion was that spirituality is an area of need for everyone, and as such deserves effective and appropriate care.

Karen Poole BN (Hons) RN (Adult)
PhD Student, Department of Nursing Research, University of Wales College of Medicine, Cardiff

Every nurse can tell the story of their first 'bed bath', that moment when you are actually expected to touch a stranger. Personally, I found the whole experience embarrassing and disturbing, as my diary at the time records:

'. . . I can't believe it, I actually had to wash this man today, it was horrible, I didn't know where to look. It wasn't just weird, it was bizarre, me washing someone my Granddad's age. I don't think I shall ever get used to this . . .'

Three years later, the embarrassment that was then so acute has ebbed away. My uniform, which at first barely disguised my novice status, has become my 'professional guise', legitimizing my actions. Becoming a 'professional nurse' seems to include possessing a 'licence to intrude'. The concept of personal space captured my imagination; a phenomenon that was invisible, yet could provoke intense emotional reactions. Just observing the way in which people in hospital seemingly marked out their territory with personal paraphernalia convinced me that this was a topic that nurses had failed to adequately discuss. As I explored the literature on the subject it became apparent that the process of concept analysis would simultaneously clarify and demonstrate the phenomenon of personal space. I hope that I have achieved this objective.

I graduated from the University of Wales College of Medicine in 1994, and was awarded a medical scholarship that is allowing me to pursue full-time doctoral studies. For 12 months, I managed to work part time as a staff nurse within the surgical directorate in the University Hospital of Wales Healthcare Trust. I now maintain my skills by supervising other BN students on their clinical placement, witnessing *their* use of personal space.

Kim Smith BSc (Hons) RGN RM
Staff Midwife, Neonatal Intensive Care Unit, Princess Anne Hospital, Southampton

I undertook general nurse training at Southampton University Hospitals qualifying as a Registered General Nurse in 1986. Prior to commencing midwifery training in 1989, I gained experience as a staff nurse on an acute medical ward. Since qualifying as a midwife I have specialized in neonatal care, completing ENB 405 – Special and Intensive Care of the Newborn, in 1991. In 1994 I completed a 4-year part-time Bachelor of Science degree course in Nursing and Midwifery, graduating with honours. A major component of this course was to undertake a research study.

My choice of topic was determined by my long-standing interest in infant comfort and infant/parental bonding. During my experience as a neonatal nurse, I became increasingly aware of the limited physical contact inevitably experienced by parents of sick or premature infants. A previous study I had carried out demonstrated that parental touch does not always have a positive effect on the physiological status of sick/premature infants. The research undertaken into 'kangaroo' care sought to explore a form of contact between infant and parent that would not have a negative effect on the infant's physiological status, while being a positive experience for the care giver.

1 Research

SECTION CONTENTS

1. Laughing at death: the ultimate paradox   3

2. Skin-to-skin contact for premature and sick infants and their mothers   31

3. The readability of patient information   79

4. Patients' and nurses' experiences of feeding: a phenomenological study   113

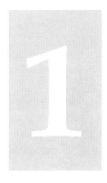

Laughing at death: the ultimate paradox

The use of humour by staff working in palliative care

Catriona Knight

Commentary

Although it has been found that the use of humour in a variety of health care settings can be a very effective intervention, it is a complex issue, perhaps even more so when that setting is palliative care.

'Black humour', 'sick humour' and similar phrases suggest an ambivalence in our attitudes towards what can be accepted and funny. Whilst we generally accept that humour should not be exploitative and derogatory, we are still unclear when humour is appropriate and when it is not. Nursing care of the dying patient demands enormous sensitivity and respect for the dignity of patients and carers. Nevertheless, to ignore the fact that humanity also includes humour is, in itself, to deny personhood. What then of nurses' humour in the context of palliative care? Is it a safety valve, an indicator of a coping strategy or is there something more profound to be explored? Is it crazy to be funny in the face of dying and death? Or is it human?

In this paper, the use of humour by nursing staff working in palliative care is very sensitively explored in what should be considered an important study.

Catriona Knight attempts to define humour, explores the potential physiological and psychosocial effects and benefits of humour and the associated research, and then proceeds to describe a grounded theory study that she performed in order to explore how nurses working in palliative care used and viewed humour.

The significant themes or core categories that emerged from data analysis were that nurses used humour as a coping mechanism, that it needed to be appropriate, related to the type and context of the humour. It was found that humour was used as a coping and stress relieving mechanism and that working in palliative care created its own brand of humour that, because of its sensitivity, would or could not be used in any other kind of setting.

Such a use of humour has been labelled 'thanatological' by Catriona. In other words it is humour related to the phenomena and practices relating to death.

This study is an excellent example of the way that grounded theory can be used to explore a nursing phenomenon and the inherently complex nature of nursing. It shows how sensitive issues can be handled in a very sensitive way, and explores what can only be regarded as a therapy with enormously powerful potential.

ABSTRACT

The complex human phenomenon of humour has been a neglected area in health care until recent years. This study aims to explore whether healthcare workers in palliative care use humour as a coping mechanism to deal with the stresses of working with the terminally ill.

A cross-section of staff working in a single National Health Service palliative care unit were interviewed using a grounded theory approach. The study attempted to extract different aspects of humour and different ways in which it is used as a coping mechanism.

There is evidence to suggest that informants did use humour as a coping mechanism and a number of themes emerged. These are discussed in relation to the literature. It also became apparent that the type of humour used in this research environment was unique. The author proposes that this unique use and style of humour is defined as 'thanatological humour'.

INTRODUCTION

It has been suggested that caring for dying people and caring for their relatives both before, during and after death is one of the most stressful situations in nursing (Farrell 1992). Many authors have alluded to humour as a method of coping. Relief theories (Darwin 1965) posited that humour released excess tension and relieved strain. It was also noted by this author that humour served not only to avoid conflict and pain, but also to express conflict and pain. Conflict theories support the idea that laughter occurs when incompatible emotions are experienced simultaneously (Pasquali 1990).

Humour is an elusive concept to define (Sumners 1990). In various European languages such as English, Polish and German, the word 'humour' carries two distinct meanings. In one sense it stands for amusing wit and in the other sense it denotes mood and a state of mind. Whether the dual meaning is purely incidental is not clear; however, the question may be asked 'Is it this duality which elicits the basic element of humour in both senses, i.e that of laughter?'. Laughter can express a certain mood, just as it may on the other hand come as response to a witty saying or act (Mishminsky 1991).

Pettifor (1982) notes that good mental health and survival in the face of adversity is dependent upon a sense of humour. Humour is thought to serve as a societal safety valve, allowing antisocial impulses to be vented harmlessly and reality to be made more tolerable (Berger 1976).

We use humour for things that we fear (Burbridge 1978, Winnick 1979), such as old age, ignorance, illness and death. When we distance ourselves from feared topics or perceive them as less powerful by laughing at them, relief is experienced (Warner 1991). It is through humour that we expand or reframe reality, which negates or diminishes the negative feelings and qualifies humour as a coping mechanism.

The great comic Charlie Chaplin succinctly stated that:

Through humour we see in what seems rational, the irrational; in what seems the important, the unimportant. It also heightens our sense of survival and preserves our sanity. It activates our sense of proportion and reveals to us in an overstatement of seriousness lurks the absurd.

(Chaplin 1966, p 226)

A REVIEW OF THE LITERATURE

The literature that dominates the nursing press has addressed the use of humour in patients and clients and how that can serve as a nursing intervention (Bellert 1989, Erdman 1991, Forsyth 1993, Hunt 1993). However, the two main areas of interest and relevance here were the relationship of humour and human physiology and the psychosocial aspects of its use. But despite all the assumptions that humour has a physiological effect on the body and psyche, knowledge of the phenomenon of humour and laughter is vague.

Literature regarding the use and benefits of humour has been noted by this author to be a neglected area until the beginning of the 1970s when the first studies of its use were beginning to appear in the medical press.

The literature is divided into two main categories, addressing the physiological effects and the psychosocial aspects of humour.

Physiological effects of humour

Historically Plato and Socrates were associated with one of the earliest theories of laughter that assumed that laughter and humour had beneficial effects on the body and mind. Medical history indicates that laughter was used as an anaesthetic for surgical procedures back in the early 13th century and in the 16th century it was used as a treatment for colds and depression. In medieval times a court jester entered the dining halls to entertain guests, since laughter was believed to aid digestion (Groves 1991). This indicates that the physiological effects of humour have long been recognized.

However, a limited degree of biological research has described the physiological process of laughter, involving neural pathways mediated by subcortical structures, especially the hypothalamus and the modulation by the cerebral cortex (Black 1984).

It has been speculated by Scott (1985) that a funny stimulus elicits an emotional response which provokes the pituitary to initiate endocrine activity leading to the production of endorphins. Endorphins are known to affect the pain threshold. Therefore laughter has a purely biological existence separate from its association with amusement.

Dugan (1989) believes there is a correlation between humour and well-being which has been recognized in the history and practice of medicine in the 20th century. Laughter and tears are believed to be the most effective of human resources for stress management. For those suffering from stress-related disorders, an inability to express oneself may result in accumulated stress which is a risk factor in heart disease, diabetes, migraine, headache and ulcerative colitis (Dugan 1989).

According to Dugan (1989), the biological function of laughter is to effect biological change – to discharge the tension that accompanies the painful emotions of fear, anger and loss. Tears and nasal secretions which are excreted during laughter contain hormones, steroids and toxins that accumulate in the body during stress (Mazer 1982).

Laughter initially stimulates the production of increased catecholamine levels in the blood. This has the effect of contracting arterial and venous musculature, which in turn increases the heart rate and elevates blood pressure. The contraction phase (sympathetic arousal) is followed by a relaxation phase (parasympathetic response) that generates a state of systemic relaxation in the organism. This may explain why some describe themselves as feeling 'pleasantly drained' after a long laugh (Scott 1985).

Dillon et al (1985) examined salivary immunogammaglobulin A (IgA) secretions and charted the daily mood of participants over a number of weeks. They stated that concentrations of salivary IgA were higher when subjects perceived their mood to be 'good' and vice versa. However, Dillon et al (1985) stated that findings are only implications and are not supported empirically. Cousins (1989) carried out a further study to look at this phenomenon by comparing IgA levels with the response from subjects after they had filled in a coping questionnaire. It was found that IgA concentrations were directly related to the subjects' perceptions of their use of humour as a coping device.

Diamond (1979) stated that laughing contracts the zygomaticus major muscle in the face, which in turn stimulates the thymus gland to secrete thymosin that regulates production of T-cell lymphocytes, contributing to a more effective immune system. Deficits in the immune system functioning following stressful events, both in animals and humans, have been noted in epidemiological studies and biophysical research to cause the immune systems to become depressed (Diamond 1979, Irwin et al 1987, Schlesinter & Yodfat 1988).

Many stressors can decrease immune system resources. Stress decreases the level of B-lymphocytes and T-lymphocytes and natural killer cells become less effective (Schlinder 1988). Haig (1988) considered that tension was released through the body via various channels, such as the viscera and motor neurons.

Laughter is aroused by pleasant thoughts and feelings that create extra nervous energy. This energy overflows into the nerves supplying the mouth and respiratory organs, causing movement and sounds associated with laughter (Diamond 1979). This was further supported by Forsyth (1993) who stated that laughter facilitates respiratory relaxation by provoking diaphragmatic breathing patterns, which are opposite patterns to emotional tensions.

Simon (1988a) recognized that claims that humour is health promoting must be substantiated by studying health outcomes. She looked at the correlation between humour and perceived health, humour and life satisfaction, and humour and morale. The results of the study show significant positive correlations between situational humour and perceived health and between situational humour and morale. Simon is one of the few authors who has entered into the quest for empirical evidence of the effect of humour on health outcomes.

Groves (1991) states that this quest is only part of the picture. Health outcomes from humour also must be researched through investigations of the correlations with the immune system, which will give greater empirical support of humour.

Many of the articles on humour are based on anecdotal evidence (Cousins 1989, Haig 1988, Scott 1985), which highlights that until recent years there has been little empirical scientific proof as to the physiological effects of humour.

Psychosocial aspects of humour

The review of the literature on humour in the psychosocial context reveals three main factors. Firstly that humour creates common ground, secondly that humour affects emotions by transferring negative emotions into positive ones, and thirdly that humour serves as a coping mechanism and relieves stress (Cousins 1983, Hunt 1993). Many authors allude to the fact that humour does have a role in stress management and in social interaction between people (Pasquali 1990, Wheaton 1983).

However, much of the evidence is anecdotal and little research has been undertaken to substantiate these notions (Hunt 1993). Despite this, attitudes toward humour as a teaching strategy and the use of humour to improve communication have been studied in an empirical manner, but overall healthcare professionals have neglected the area (Sumners 1990). Much of the literature focuses on healthcare professionals and the use of humour with clients, but little reference is made to humour as a coping mechanism for staff.

Laughter and tears are useful in stress management to reduce social and emotional distance among people and groups (Dugan 1989). In social settings shared laughter 'breaks the ice', facilitating emotional contact with a group of people. In healthcare settings, where access to emotionally supportive humans is available, this acts as a major source of stress management (Matthews-Simonton 1984). Shared laughter can have the same effect even among strangers. Robinson (1977) stated that humour helps to relieve stress, anxiety, hostility and aggression in a socially acceptable way.

Parse (1993) examined the role of laughter in human health and stated that it carries various positive meanings, for example feelings of togetherness, closeness, warmth and friendliness.

In her theory 'Man-Living-Health' (now Human Becoming), Parse (1993) associates experiences of humour with experiences of health. Malinsky (1991) makes the same connection on the basis of Rogers' science of unitary human beings.

Cousins (1989) stated that humour is a way in which we can express our humility. By joining in humour and acknowledging our oneness, we have profound expectations of unity and co-operation and he views it as enfolding the other person in caring, understanding and support. This view is supported by Dugan

(1989), who stated that bringing more laughter and humour into the workplace itself helps to maintain and develop social support and nurturing systems. According to Kubie (1971), humour is a social lubricant, easing certain types of shyness and tension. It acts as a resource for informal staff support that occurs throughout the work day (Killeen 1991) and it can aid communication (Metcalf 1987, Robinson 1977, Rosenheim & Golan 1986).

Much of this literature supports the view that humour is used to facilitate communication. It can be shared (Bellert 1989) and establishes a rapport and communication which conveys emotional messages (Robinson 1977).

Smith Lee (1990) stated that laughing together unites people because it shows acceptance of others and creates a common bond. It is viewed as akin to sharing a meal or other pleasurable event. Laughter is a contagious, social experience which has a cohesive effect on human beings.

However, Rosenburg (1989) stated that some people take themselves and their environment seriously. Humour is not therefore a significant part of their day-to-day relationships, but the author continues to state that at some point in life, everyone has used humour or sarcasm to help deal with something unpleasant or to cope with an event until ready to take an indepth look at the situation. This may be viewed as avoidance tactics.

The benefits and rationale for developing humorous attitudes in people facing serious, often life-threatening illness are appearing with increasing frequency in the literature (Herth 1990, Killeen 1991). Laughing in the face of death enables healthcare professionals to confront a taboo subject and rob it of some of its mysterious hold (Klein 1986).

Humour strategies can create a more comfortable work environment (Smith Lee 1990). Although it was demonstrated that humour can improve attendance, attitude and productivity, there was no reference to other supportive material.

Vaillant (1977) refers to humour as one of the most elegant of the defence mechanisms. It may be logical to assume that humour is a survival skill.

Another author reported that 'Humour has the potential to be a valuable communication tool available to the therapist in furthering insight, monitoring dynamic states, and catalyzing higher levels of the adaptive process . . .' (Hickson 1977, p 66).

Staff have been noted to use humour as a way of dealing with the day-to-day stress of nursing (Hutchinson 1987, Leiber 1986).

Warner (1991) undertook a descriptive study which looks at the circumstances under which student nurses chose to use humour as a coping mechanism, as well as describing how they chose humour to cope with intrapersonal and interpersonal threats. It concludes that students use cognitive, appraisal and humorous coping to mediate the stressful person–environment relationships for positive outcomes. This supports some of the anecdotal reports stating that humour serves as a coping mechanism for healthcare professionals. Warner (1991) stated that humour can be used as a healthy catharsis, which supports the idea that humour serves as a stress release and coping strategy.

In conclusion, as previously stated, in the field of health care there has been little precise research on the use of and value of humour. However, humour is an issue that warrants more serious attention and the work so far may be enhanced by quantitative and qualitative approaches that will shed further light on this intriguing phenomenon.

THE RESEARCH

Humour is an elusive concept to define (Sumners 1990). Because humour is such a subjective concept the author felt that it was not appropriate to use quantitative techniques as these methods rely heavily on acquiring data that are numerical and statistically interpreted.

Leininger (1985) stated that the 'social world' does not lend itself to the forms of objective measurement which are synonymous with quantitative research. The study of people requires us to, as Melia (1982) stated, 'tell it as it is'.

Qualitative methodology is primarily concerned with the in-depth study of human phenomena, as it allows the researcher to explore the meanings of events and processes for the people who are experiencing them. This is also supported by Polit & Hungler (1985), who state that qualitative research typically involves the collection and analysis of loosely structured information regarding people in their naturalistic setting, which is the aim of this study. Qualitative research is especially well suited to description, hypothesis generation and theory development.

Qualitative research processes are able to 'bring alive' particular situations and people under study and these approaches are advocated where there is little or no literature on the notion being studied, when it is a new area of knowledge (Leininger 1985).

Six informants consented to be interviewed. The informants represented one of the disciplines of either trained nurse, un-trained nurse, physiotherapist, occupational therapist, social worker and doctor.

Semistructured interview was used and field notes taken throughout. A tape recorder was used and the interviews were transcribed in full in order to interpret as fully as possible the totality of what is being studied.

The transcriptions were analysed to search for themes using constant comparison, by comparing the categories and redefining theoretically relevant categories from data previously collected. The theory was developed around core categories. These categories were further divided into subcategories.

This research aimed to uphold the key principles issued by the Royal College of Nursing (1977), which are informed consent, freedom from harm, and anonymity and confidentiality.

DATA ANALYSIS

Three main themes emerged from the analysis of the interviews. The first theme is humour as a coping mechanism, the second is the appropriateness of humour and the third is the type and context of humour in the workplace. They are further broken down into subcategories.

Humour as a coping mechanism

Throughout the interviews the use of humour as a coping mechanism emerged and was taken as a significant theme. It was further broken down into subcategories:

1. emotional release
2. physical effects
3. mood alteration
4. avoidance.

Emotional release

The literature reveals that humour has been recognized as a way of expressing difficult or painful emotions (McHale 1989). All of the informants described humour, by their definition, as a release. As one informant stated:

> ... the relief you sort of get when you physically sigh ... you know when you breathe out, you sigh about something, you get that releasing feeling I get when I laugh ... like an emotional explosion that's enjoyable.

All of the informants at some point in the interview used euphemisms to describe the emotional release of humour.

> . . . it lightens my step, I bounce instead of dragging my feet.

Only a few of the informants actually used the word 'coping' or a derivative. For example, '. . . humour is a coping mechanism or an abreaction [sic] to release the . . . er . . . emotion'. One of the informants did not necessarily view humour as a way of coping with the job that they do, but as a facing up to their own death.

> . . . everyone has a problem coping with death, particularly their own death.

The concept of coping with one's own death was evident in some of the informants' replies.

> . . . sharing laughter or a joke about a situation one has . . . er . . . found difficult and made you look at your own death, it helps you cope with death, particularly your own . . . the time when you think, by the grace of God go I.

Another informant then went on to describe why the need to find a coping strategy was required, stating:

> . . . you can't do much about the fact that you are going to die . . .
> helping you as an individual to come to terms with it, is partly
> to make a joke about it, because it is so, so horrific, the thought
> is so horrendous really, it is one of the ways we struggle with it
> really.

Warner (1991) states that situations that evoke painful emotions result in the use of cognitive coping strategies, which included minimizing the event by using humour to allow healthcare workers to regulate stressful emotions.

It was strongly acknowledged that the nature of their work created the need to deal with some of the painful emotions it raised. Mishminsky (1991) states that humour is one of the 'struggle tactics' where people can confront and deal with some of the painful emotions and anxiety in dealing with death. This was also supported by an informant:

> . . . it helps you deal with the bad things, a way of bringing them out, otherwise you could quite easily keep them in your mind and not let go of them.

And another suggested that failure to express emotion could have a detrimental effect on coping with other stresses.

> . . . if you don't deal with some of the painful things that this kind of job presents you with, you can't go on to help the next person, having a good laugh shifts some of the pain.

A similar belief is held by Rosenburg (1989) who states that nurses and clinicians use black comedy as a way of preventing burnout.

Physical effects

Humour has been found to have demonstrable effects on several body systems, including stimulating the release of hormones into the vascular system (Dillon et al 1985). All of the informants stated that they found the physical effects of humour difficult to articulate, by stating that:

. . . I don't know if I could name them . . . it's difficult to say what's happening inside . . .

. . . it's difficult to say exactly how I feel.

. . . it's really hard to say what's going on physically when you laugh although . . . when you . . . er think about it . . . something is happening.

~ They stated that despite the difficulty in defining it, there was some kind of physical effect.

. . . it does affect you physically when you stop and think about it.

. . . I think also that it is a physical response.

. . . It's also a physical release really, you know it's er . . . er . . . it's like being able to . . . the relief you sort of get when you physically sigh . . . you know when you breathe out, that's the sort of feeling I get when I laugh.

The physical responses described can be further divided into physiological responses and responses of a more subjective nature, such as relaxation.

. . . if I do laugh I get a gut ache [laughs] if I really laugh I do, it means that I'm laughing too much.

. . . It can make your ribs hurt and your belly . . . I suppose that is why we call it belly laughing [laughs].

The facial, chest, abdominal and skeletal muscles involved in the gastrointestinal system are stimulated during laughter (Bellert 1989).

Groves (1991) states that humour physiologically stimulates the cardiac and respiratory system, increasing the cardiac load and respiratory demand and effort. Despite the informants describing feelings of relaxation, they also contradict Mazer's (1982) theory of relaxation which presents empirical evidence which suggests that respiratory relaxation is achieved through laughter.

... you realize that your heart rate shoots up ... you can also feel that you are never ever going to take a breath again [laughs].

... laughing a lot can make you feel quite breathless ...

However, the examples the informants gave of physical relaxation are well documented in the literature (Dugan 1989, Groves 1991, Sumners 1990).

Dugan (1989) states that tranquilizers and muscle relaxants help patients achieve physiological relaxation. He believes that laughter often produces the same beneficial results as medications, chiefly a physiological relaxation response. This anecdotal assumption is supported by Mazer (1982) who stated that increased catecholamine levels in the blood stimulate other measurable physiological responses, which in turn generate a state of systemic relaxation in the organism.

... when there is a bit of humour in the group people relax I think ...

... difficult to say exactly how I feel ... um ... you're relaxed, the tension goes ...

... But, yes, tension, if you do reduce the tension then it is more relaxing.

Dugan (1989) stated that this response explains why people feel 'pleasantly drained' after laughing.

... it can make you feel really tired, because ... because, well ... I suppose you use a lot of energy don't you?

... It's very physical when you laugh ... every part of you moves and you gasp for air and hold your stomach muscles because they hurt so much ... [laughs].

Mood alteration

Humour has been reported to affect the mood (Rosenburg 1989). Some informants stated that the mood effect of humour is a positive one.

... the general feeling that it gives you will stay, the emotional physical feeling is short-lived. The emotional feeling ... the up it gives you will last longer.

... a good laugh does make you feel better ... I suppose that it does alter mood.

... When I laugh at something that really tickles me, it puts me in a better mood and I don't seem to get so wound up about the next person.

Siegel (1986) stated that humour's most important function is to jolt individuals out of their habitual frame of mind to create new perspectives. Some of the informants' responses did not reflect this notion.

> ... If you are feeling really low and wallowing in misery, people laughing around you can make you feel worse ... you feel ... you feel ... that you can laugh at the time but when all the humour disappears the problem is still with you ... it won't just disappear into thin air.

> ... If you are laughing at something that someone is feeling sensitive about, you can put them into a really bad mood and make them feel worse.

This does not support Smith Lee's (1990) notion that it is almost impossible to have a good laugh and feel bad at the same time.

Warner (1991) believed that laughter is a behavioural expression of an internal state in which negative effects and tensions are replaced by positive effects and relief. Some of the informants' replies supported this belief.

> ... you can feel pretty down when you have had to deal with sad people, but if you can laugh about something, you can feel better and go home in a better mood instead of feeling really low and scratchy.

However, this is supported by Forsyth (1993) who purports that if humour is applied inadvertently, it has the potential to wreak undue damage which could have long-lasting effects.

> ... If you are depressed you don't see anything as very funny really, everything seems black, so maybe when your mood is low, certainly as an individual the humour has gone really ... for a time.

Mishminsky (1991) stated that the main thing is the intention of humour, whether it is reacting in relation to oneself or other people.

Avoidance

Avoidance of painful situations and feelings has long been acknowledged as a valid coping mechanism. Avoidance is a form of denial which, according to Campbell (1981), is generally conceived as a means of disowning the existence of unpleasant reality. Denial or avoidance is the most common element in a variety of defences that involve either conscious or unconscious repudiation of events in order to decrease anxiety and other unpleasant side-effects (Weisman & Hackett 1961).

Working in palliative care has already been shown to be a high stress occupation. All of the informants acknowledged that their role in caring for the terminally ill and dying was emotionally stressful.

. . . I think that it can have an accumulative effect . . . I think that if you have one death you know, it's tough . . . but, you know you talk about it, it's the accumulation of all of the deaths that you have to avoid, so you don't get yourself . . . really drowned . . . the small sadness that builds up.

. . . The job we have to do here can be traumatic and of great personal emotional expense.

. . . it can be very emotionally draining . . . sometimes you feel as if you have been dragged through an emotional hedge backwards.

. . . it's stopping real things happening by making jokes of it . . .

. . . that is quite . . . can be quite painful, it is an easier way in which to discuss it by being, flip, then you can discuss . . . it, without the . . . pain.

The coping mechanism of avoidance is supported by Bellert (1989) who states that one of the purposes of humour is that it allows a temporary escape from reality.

Avoidance of emotional involvement was found to be a reason to use humour for some informants.

. . . survival is this business of detachment, not to get emotionally involved and using humour avoids . . . er . . . this kind of overinvolvement with clients.

. . . you have to be able to call it a day if you see what I mean . . . because it is so emotionally taxing and painful you have to make light of things and avoid analysing the real truth behind a situation.

Forsyth (1993) stated that humour may be used to deny the seriousness of problems, mask feelings and avoid dealing with important and pertinent issues.

Detachment from real emotions was a reason put forward by some informants as to why humour is used.

. . . it's almost because you can't bear to think about them and what's happening around you.

. . . if we took on the grief that we deal with we would be nervous wrecks . . . we have to . . . be able to put the feeling away. I suppose humour does that really . . . you know . . . all that hidden pain . . . it helps you express it . . . without having to deal with the real problem . . .

Appropriateness of humour

Throughout the interview the area of appropriateness of humour was explored by the informants. This was further broken down into subcategories:

1. normalization and comfort

2. situational
3. acceptability.

Normalization and comfort

Attitudes towards humour are based on belief systems and are influenced by learning and also in the feedback of others' approval (Sumners 1990). It is evident that the informants faced some personal discomfort when humour is used.

... at times you realize that you are being incredibly obscure, because other people are recognizing it as being funny too. So you don't tend to think oh crikey, that's me going off my trolley, you recognize that other people are seeing it as humorous as well.

... we are all oddpots really.

... sometimes you feel ... er ... others are thinking why has she found this so funny? But then you realize that they think that it is funny too ... you almost rely on others' laughter to feel what you are laughing about is OK.

... I think that I'm really ... really warped when I laugh at others' misfortune, but on the other hand you have to realize that it's not really being cruel because everyone is doing it and you're not being ... being directly unkind to the patient.

It became evident that informants did not feel that they should or would pass judgement on the type of humour being used.

... you shouldn't feel judged on what you find humorous ...

And another informant stated:

... I don't expect people to tick me off for laughing about something unless I was being totally indiscreet or something, likewise I wouldn't, definitely not do it to someone else ...

Situational

Sumners (1990) viewed humour as a positive force in professional practice settings when it is used judiciously and with knowledge and discretion. Some informants stated that to use humour which they regarded as appropriate required some modification to the timing of their open appreciation of a humorous situation.

... sometimes I have to laugh inwardly about a situation ... sometimes you could be talking to somebody and something could be happening and you're absolutely desperate to laugh, but you know that it wouldn't be appropriate at that time, but having said that you can laugh about it later.

... I think that there are times to laugh and times when not to laugh . . . there are times when people feel, have a general feeling when to be sober about it because there are certain people around or certain situations when it wouldn't be appropriate to be rolling around in laughter.

It was also felt that if a situation should arise and the humour was inappropriate then much of the humour and its benefits would be negated.

. . . if you laugh at a time which you know to be inappropriate, you can feel really bad and you don't find it so, so funny, I think . . . I think that is because you feel silly or childish and that you have possibly made someone feel hurt or uncomfortable . . . you have to be very careful on the whole.

. . . when something is very tense . . . you can break it with something very funny and people will respond as long as it's not unkind, not at anyone's expense.

. . . it's a terrible feeling when you really want to laugh at something and you know that you can't . . . not just the suppression of the laughter but also you realize that it could get you into trouble . . . so it's quite worrying when that happens.

Another discussed the appropriateness of humour in a crisis situation.

. . . It's a case of if you don't laugh you would cry in a crisis situation, then the whole place would fall apart, so the right person needs the right something to drop in. I haven't got a sense of humour [laughs], I really haven't.

Acceptability

It was suggested that before humour became acceptable in an environment, permission had to be sought.

. . . You have to look at if everyone has the same potential for humour before you have the authority or permission to be humorous in the way that we are here.

. . . So there is something about appropriateness, you almost need permission to find something funny.

There also needs to be discretion over whom you were sharing the humour with.

. . . it has to be . . . acceptable . . . there is a component of taste and what's acceptable to one person may not be acceptable to another.

. . . you can't share a joke or a funny situation with anyone. You have to assess their situation and how they will perceive the joke.

It had also been stated that there had been occasions where humour had caused distress to visiting healthcare professionals.

... people were making a joke about a chap that only had five minutes to live, er, I can see that it wasn't entirely appropriate, they have rather a high view of doctors, and that kind of fooling around was, that was how it was seen.

Humour was not always appropriate in the context of personal experience and life events.

... if you are feeling a bit sensitive about something ... say for example my mother had reached the terminal stages of cancer, I think that it can be very upsetting and people need to think carefully, just a bit more sensitively to the people they are sharing things with.

Killeen (1991) stated that laughing about a problem can overcome the psychological barriers that surround it. However, it may be suggested that receiving others' humour about a painful personal aspect is not the person's own perspective, but something forced upon them by others.

Humour in the work environment

From the interviews emerged a unique type of humour used in the researched environment. This was taken as a significant theme and further broken down into two categories:

1. type of humour used
2. contextual.

Type of humour used

Humour means something different to everyone (Mishminsky 1991). Some informants used humour for the things that they feared and to avoid the things they found painful. All of the informants stated that they used black humour. The *Concise Oxford Dictionary* (1982), defines black humour as 'a presentation of tragedy or bitter reality in comic terms'.

... definitely black humour, what one would expect from a place like this ... we wouldn't laugh very much if we waited for the good things that happened to patients.

... Sometimes we can be really sick here, it's difficult to define I expect it surpasses the realms of black humour ... [laughs] it is probably more macabre and give the psychologists a field day [more laughter].

Mishminsky (1991) states that humour is here to assert itself against the unkindness of real circumstances, 'we laugh at the things we fear'.

Some informants were specific as to the type of circumstances or events that they found funny.

. . . they were able to laugh and joke about death and everyone has a problem coping with their own death and so on . . .

. . . we do a slot on death . . . a joke about a chap that's only got five minutes to live.

. . . it's humour that's connected with er . . . subjects like death and dying.

An extract from the transcriptions exemplifies that type of humour.

. . . Somebody from Homecare went on holiday with their niece, they went abroad on a coach, they were very frail and we were really quite concerned about them and how they were going to manage, they went by coach all round France, Austria and Germany and they came back and they were dead [laughter over dialogue] in the coach when they arrived back in Southampton [more laughter] . . . and, and, we thought that was wonderful she actually got a holiday . . . [further laughter over dialogue] we felt pretty sorry for the coach driver, we thought it was an absolute scream [further laughter] that this lady got all the way round, had a holiday, really enjoyed it . . . but was actually dead when she got back [more laughter]. If you said to someone outside that this lady actually died on the way back [more laughter] they would be horrified. They would say how awful, what a shame you know. And for us, we say, well she got a holiday anyway, thank goodness she didn't die at the beginning of it, you know, she had her priorities right.

Killeen (1991) stated that healthcare professionals use black comedy and sarcasm as avoidance techniques.

. . . to the greatest part quite black and secondary probably sarcastic . . . and following that probably just fun.

Humour in this context is stated to have other functions also.

. . . I might be looking for an opportunity to shut them up . . . and [laughs] and humour might be a good way of breaking other people's er . . . chain of thought.

. . . I think physical activities . . . like squirting people with water.

Humour has positive and negative facets (Bellert 1989).

. . . I think that humour can be used to humiliate people probably too.

. . . in a sense it's making fun out of people really.

. . . you have to exercise a little caution, I've seen humour used to ridicule and humiliate people, saying that . . . I really haven't seen it here . . . really, no.

Despite acknowledgement that humour could be used to humiliate people, informants clarified the belief that they did not actually cause harm to the patient or others.

. . . it could be used to hurt people, but because of the type of humour

we have to be very, very careful where we say it . . . and to
who . . . walls have ears you know [laughs].

Therefore the data reveal that there are four main aspects
of humour that are used in the chosen setting. Evidence as to
the type of humour can be seen in extracts lifted from the transcriptions of humorous incidents and jokes that informants used
to illustrate a point.

. . . We were in the Round the other day . . . one of the patients an
elderly chap [laughs] was under discussion. This chap was profoundly
deaf and couldn't speak properly [laughs over dialogue] the funny
thing was that he had refused to come into XXXX, because his blind,
elderly sister, with whom he lived, had been in hospital following a
heart attack [laughs more] . . . the reason he wanted to delay the
admission was because he had some money and a Will which was
hidden under the floorboard, which his sister needed to be able to
find . . . I think that he thought XXXX was his last port of call [laughs].
Everyone found that really amusing how a deaf mute man wanted to
tell a blind lady where to find his Will and money [further laughter],
we laughed about that for ages trying to come up with some idiotic
solutions to the problem [laughter interspersed with dialogue], it was
really unkind if you think about it.

There has to be a degree of acceptability as to the type of
humour before it can be used out of the specific workplace.
Therefore it may be proposed that the type of humour is particular and unique to the researched environment.

. . . There is a lot of unsaid stuff, you can make a comment and you
don't need to say any more than that, like in Plymouth when patients
bleed to death they give them red towels, so that . . . that sounds
disgusting [laughter over dialogue accompanied by researcher restricting the ability to speak] so if I ever get a red towel [laughter restricting
the ability to speak], I'll know that I am about to bleed to death . . .
[more laughter] . . . I can't believe it . . . I would rather have a white
towel that went red and not know anything about it . . . it's so it's not
apparent how much people have lost . . . I think that is really gross . . .

Contextual

Some informants felt that they would not use the same type of
humour in a different environment.

. . . you certainly wouldn't use sick type of humour in every situation
and I'm often, you know, the times when you use laughter a lot, sick
jokes here, you certainly wouldn't use this humour in any other setting
[laughs].

. . . now in other areas that I have worked there hasn't been nearly as
much humour there . . . as there is here . . . whether that indicates that
this environment warrants that more humour takes place for other
coincidental reasons . . . I don't know . . . I would hazard a guess that

people . . . actually enjoy it here as a way of dealing with what we actually do.

Some informants, although they did not mention other work environments, stated that the type of humour used in this particular establishment was 'in house' and felt that it could not be used out of this context.

Forsyth (1993) stated that the incongruity and developmental theories of humour stress absurd, unexpected, inappropriate or out-of-context events as a basis for humour. Such incongruous events can alternatively result in anxiety and therefore the perception of humour is dependent upon how the incongruity is understood in the context in which it occurs.

. . . the other person may not be an 'in' person, but there seems to be less humour . . . maybe that's because there is an outsider . . . and obviously your presence may disrupt the, the dynamics . . .

. . . not part of the unit, not part of the team, so 'in' jokes are, which are very funny to those who work here, are not so funny to those who are from the outside.

Some informants described the effect of using workplace humour on outsiders or those who did not work within this particular unit.

. . . when we had the review, we had it every Christmas . . . one year the volunteers were terribly upset by it, but the staff thought it was hilarious. It was just too serious for the others . . .

. . . so you wouldn't do it with anyone outside. I wouldn't make jokes about death to anyone outside our group, it has to be . . . within.

. . . you can fall about laughing, but anyone who didn't work here would think that it is totally unsuitable to be laughing at.

Others described the effect of using 'in house' humour at home.

. . . I have used it in a home situation er . . . er . . . home people are a bit sort of gobsmacked by it . . . a bit near the bone.

. . . I made the mistake of telling a little joke to some friends at home . . . or should I say ex-friends [laughs] about a little amusing incident . . . I was the only one laughing and I felt ostracized for the rest of the evening.

A reason was offered as to why outsiders may find the described humour offensive.

. . . it's almost as if we have taken the blatant sensitivity out of the tragic situations, outsiders can't detach themselves from the grim reality . . . I . . . I suppose that they don't have to, do they?

Another used an analogy to explain why others may find the humour offensive.

... If I heard jokes about slaughter houses and how the animals were and what they did ... I would have a total sense of humour failure, it would really upset me because I don't understand it and work with it.

An informant summarized the thoughts and feelings of the others.

... I wouldn't now tell people what kind of things we laugh at ... it's something special and only for those who really understand the nature of our work ... and the fact that we are all basically kind people really ... I suppose.

Informants speculated that humour was used as a coping mechanism in order to reduce anxiety to a level where death is manageable to that person.

... to bring it down to a level that you can actually cope with.

... because we see so much pain and suffering it helps to bring the sadness down to a level where it is manageable.

DISCUSSION

The main themes that have emerged from this study are as follows:

1. Humour is used in this setting as a coping mechanism.
2. Humour alleviates stress by altering the mood of the individual or environment in which it is used.
3. The type of humour used in this setting is seen by the author as unique to the researched environment.

A standard dictionary definition states that humour is:

the ability of a person to see when things are amusing, rather than being serious all the time; the way that a particular person or group of people is amused by certain things but not by others, and a quality in something that makes one laugh, for example in a situation, in someone's words or actions, or in a book or film (*Collins Dictionary* 1987).

Humour is a complex phenomenon and various definitions have been developed. Simon (1988b) believed humour refers to a mood or state of mind in a person that is conducive to producing laughter and fun. Parse (1993) has studied the role of laughter in human health and says that it carries various positive meanings, such as togetherness and friendliness.

Astedt-Kurki & Liukkonen (1994) stated that humour is a personal and individual matter. Although there is evidence in other literature to support this statement, in this study it has become evident that humour within palliative care is predominantly of a specific type, being 'black' humour. It is evident that the humour used within this context is very specific. It is noted that none of the informants would use the type of humour described in other settings. There is very little literature available on the relevance of the type of humour used or its significance in the palliative care setting.

Humour can be classed as a type in itself and does not fall into any category that has previously been defined. It is noted that the humour used is beyond what has been defined as black or gallows humour, but may more suitably be described by the author as 'thanatological' humour, with 'thanatology' being defined as the phenomena accompanying practices relating to death, from the Greek word *thanos* meaning death (*Concise Oxford Dictionary* 1982). This has been chosen because much of the humour used is about people who are terminally ill.

It is suggested that the very reason this type of humour is used directly relates to the very thing that the informants have acknowledged to be stressful and likely to cause personal discomfort if not managed adequately by employing effective coping strategies.

Many of the informants believed that the type and use of their humour was atypical in comparison to their experience gained in other settings. The cause of this discomfort and the quest to be reassured that this use of humour is acceptable may stem from the fact that nursing generally is seen as a caring profession. Dying and terminal illness are generally perceived as sad events and earn respect because of their nature, inherent in Western society's beliefs and values. Laughter has been thought of as mocking those who are less fortunate or have a life-affecting disorder or circumstances (Groves 1991).

The thought of these beliefs and values together may create in the individual cognitive dissonance. When laughter was experienced coupled with the previously stated Western values it is noted that this may have resulted in incongruity of effect. It may be suggested from the data that, as a result of cognitive dissonance and incongruity of effect, informants seek approval by observing individuals for their use of humour and the response to their own use of humour.

The incongruity and developmental theories of humour stress absurd, unexpected, inappropriate, or out-of-context events as a basis for humour (Forsyth 1993). There is evidence from the transcriptions to suggest that the type of humour is very much in the context of that environment and would be inappropriate in another situation. It is possible that because of this incongruity of effect, humour may give rise to feelings of guilt.

Sumners (1990) believed that attitudes towards humour are based on the approval of others. The data suggest that when taking the type of humour out of the researched context, the informants felt that there would be disapproval from others who did not understand the very nature of this working environment. Such incongruous events may alternatively result in anxiety and therefore perception of humour is dependent upon how the incongruity is understood in the context in which it occurs.

Most informants did not feel able to share this type of humour in another environment, be it at home or in another work situation. Although some informants did not verbalize feelings of guilt associated with the use of humour, from the transcriptions and recordings it may have been suggested since there was ambivalence and hesitancy in the replies. This may indicate that there was conflict in their feelings regarding the use of such types of humour and as previously stated, this may cause anxiety. The humour used is unique to the informants' workplace and may not be deemed 'socially acceptable' outside this environment.

The effects of humour on mood have been well documented. This may be because the work in palliative care can be emotionally demanding. The data suggest that the informants did experience a change in mood when using humour. The most noted change in mood was a positive one. This may be related to the concept that humour serves as a coping mechanism by altering mood and hence the ability to reframe reality. This supports previous findings by Jaffe & Scott (1984).

Humour has been noted to serve as a coping mechanism in other areas of work or stress. Not only has it been noted for its cognitive effect but also for physiological changes that take place with humour and laughter, despite a lack of empirical evidence.

It was noted that humour was used as a coping mechanism by avoiding having to deal with situations that caused discomfort and fear. Campbell (1981) believed that avoidance is a form of denial that enables a person to disown the existence of an unpleasant reality. It may be debated that humour in this form may be beneficial or detrimental to the psychological health of the informants. Denial may be a form of repression and an inability to deal with the stark reality of a painful situation.

This is supported by Forsyth (1993), who mooted that humour may serve to deny the seriousness of the problem and to avoid dealing with important and pertinent issues. This repression may have detrimental effects on the individual. It is suggested from the data that cognitive coping strategies are used by the informants to negate the unpleasant emotions, including distancing from, rising above and minimizing the event, escalating the situation to the absurd, using what Warner (1991) called 'cognitive shifts and mastery'.

This may raise the questions 'when does the use of humour become a maladaptive mechanism of defence? Or is denial maladaptive at all?'. Lazarus (1980) supports the adaptive role of denial in the discussion on stress and suggests that stress is viewed as an occurring transaction between the environment and the person. Since some stressors are unchangeable, for example terminal disease, denial in the form of humour can be seen as an appropriate coping tool, lessening the stressful effect.

This is also supported by Mishminsky (1991) who stated that every humorous thought must be based on both reason and absurdity. This appears to be the essential dialectic of humour in this situation.

This supports the findings that humour, above and beyond any other use, is a valid and dependable coping strategy for the researched environment.

Although physiological effects have been measured the author notes that informants were largely unaware of or unable to quantify any physiological changes taking place during or after what they regarded as a 'good laugh'.

Healthcare professionals need to find coping mechanisms to prevent the negative effects of a high stress occupation (Hutchinson 1987). The informants felt that humour served more than one function, but predominantly that of dealing with emotional pain and its effect on altering mood. However, it has to be acknowledged that humour cannot serve as a panacea to all discomforts (Sumners 1990).

Humour may be used because it allows expression of stressful events without a person being seen as a non-coper. Often direct acknowledgement of stresses and difficulties has been perceived by others to be a sign of weakness (Bond 1986).

Humour has emerged throughout this study as having a significant role in the everyday function of staff and the dynamics of the establishment. There is little evidence from the data that the concept of humour as coping mechanism is not acknowledged by the informants' colleagues. It is suggested that the reason may be the need to avoid breaking down the psychological barriers and the need to be regarded as a 'coper'.

Interestingly, no difference between the type of humour used by the different disciplines was apparent from the data.

The data suggest that the type of humour used in this setting is unique and can be described as 'thanatological'. This may suggest that it is the context and experience of working with the terminally ill that elicits 'thanotological' humour rather than their role within that setting.

CONCLUSIONS

Humour has emerged from this study as a mechanism by which employees in this particular setting cope with the demands of their role within the team. The data suggest that strategies are required by healthcare workers to reduce the stress created by this environment. Humour has been noted to reduce stress by altering mood and hence helps to reduce tension from stressful situations, especially the accumulative stress of caring for those with a life-threatening disease and approaching the terminal stage of their illness.

It is believed that healthcare workers need to acknowledge that some humour is necessary to enable them perform their role within this context. If this was achieved, it may result in a reduction of guilt associated with its use.

It is difficult to ascertain from this study whether the type of humour apparent in this researched environment is typical of other similar environments. This also raises the question as to whether the type of humour used here would occur in a different work environment.

RECOMMENDATIONS FOR FURTHER STUDY

In the light of the issues raised through this research, the following recommendations are presented for consideration.

As previously stated, it cannot be clear from this study whether humour described in this setting is unique to the researched environment. Further study of a similar nature into other healthcare environments may provide clearer insight into this phenomenon.

Many of the informants stated that they did feel some physiological change taking place with the use of humour. Perhaps further study into the physiological effect of laughter would give clearer insight as to why humour can affect mood and cognitive process. This may develop further previous scientific evidence (Dillon et al 1985, Fry 1979, Schlesinter & Yodfat 1988).

Humour has been demonstrated in other studies to have positive effects on an individual to enhance coping. In the light of this, it is recommended that humour may be used as a formal coping tool in the context of staff support. The effects of formalizing humour as a means of staff support would need to be closely evaluated to elicit whether it continues to function as a coping mechanism or whether its situational nature is the very essence of its value as a coping mechanism. This poses the question 'If humour was legitimized in this setting, would it still continue to function as a coping mechanism?'.

Acknowledgements

Thanks are extended to Mr J Warr for his support and supervision with this study and to the informants who so freely and willingly gave of their time.

REFERENCES

Astedt-Kurki P, Liukkonen A 1994 Humour in nursing care. Journal of Advanced Nursing 20: 183–188

Bellert J 1989 Humour: a therapeutic approach in oncology nursing. Cancer Nursing 12(2): 65–70

Berger A 1976 Anatomy of a joke. Journal of Communication 26(3): 113–115

Black D 1984 Laughter. Journal of the American Medical Association 252: 2995

Bond M 1986 Stress and self-awareness: a guide for nurses. Heinemann Nursing, London

Burbridge R 1978 The nature and potential of therapeutic humour. Cited in: Warner S Humour: a coping response for student nurses. Archive of Psychiatric Nursing 5(1): 10–16

Campbell R 1981 Psychiatry Dictionary, 5th edn. Oxford University Press, New York

Chaplin C 1966 My autobiography. Pocket Books, New York

Collins Dictionary 1987 W T Mcleod (ed) William Collins, Glasgow

Concise Oxford Dictionary 1982 J B Sykes (ed) Guild Publishing, London

Cousins N 1983 The healing heart. Avon, New York

Cousins N 1989 Proving the power of laughter. Psychology Today October: 1485–1493

Darwin C 1865 The expression of emotion in man. Chicago

Diamond J 1979 Your body doesn't lie. Warner, New York

Dillon K, Minchoff B, Baker R H 1985 Positive emotional states and the enhancement of the immune system. International Journal of Psychiatry in Medicine 15(1): 13–18

Dugan D 1989 Laughter and tears: best medicine for stress. Nursing Forum XXIV(1)

Erdman L 1991 Laughter therapy for patients with cancer. Oncology Nurse Forum 18(8): 1359–1363

Farrell M 1992 Process of mutual support. Professional Nurse 8(1): 10–14

Forsyth A 1993 Humour and the psychotherapeutic process. British Journal of Nursing 2: 19

Fry W Jr 1979 Humour and the cardiovascular system. In: Fry W Jr (ed) The Study of Humour. Antioch University Press, Los Angeles

Groves D 1991 A merry heart doeth good like medicine. Holistic Nursing Practice 5(4): 49–56

Haig R 1988 The anatomy of humour: biopsychosocial and therapeutic perspectives. Charles Thomas, Springfield

Herth K 1990 Contributions of humour as perceived by the terminally ill. American Journal of Hospice Care 7(1): 36–40

Hickson J 1977 Humour as an element in the counselling relationship. Psychology 14: 60–68

Hunt A 1993 Humour as a nursing intervention. Cancer Nursing 16: 1

Hutchinson S 1987 Self care and job stress. Image 19(4): 192–196

Irwin M, Daniels M, Bloom E, Smith T L, Wiener H 1987 Life events, depressive symptoms and immune function. American Journal of Psychiatry 144(4): 437–446

Jaffe D, Scott C 1984 From burnout to balance. McGraw-Hill, New York

Killeen M 1991 Clinical clowning: humour in hospice care. American Journal of Hospice and Palliative Care May/June: 23–27

Klein A 1986 Humour and death: you have got to be kidding. American Journal of Hospice Care 3(4): 42–45

Kubie L 1971 The destructive potential of humour in psychotherapy. American Journal of Psychiatry 127(7): 861–866

Lazarus R, Folkman S (eds) 1980 Stress appraisal and coping. Springer, New York

Leiber D 1986 Laughter and humour in critical care. Dimensions of Critical Care Nursing 5: 162–170

Leininger M 1985 Qualitative research methods in nursing. Grune and Stratton

Malinsky V 1991 The experience of laughing at oneself in older couples. Nursing Science Quarterly 4: 69–75

Matthews-Simonton S 1984 The healing family. Bantam, New York

Mazer 1982 10 sure-fire stress releasers. Prevention 34: 104–106

McHale M 1989 Getting the joke – interpreting humour in group therapy. Journal of Psychosocial Nursing and Mental Health Services 27(9): 24–29

Melia K 1982 'Tell it as it is' – qualitative methodology and nursing research: understanding the nurse's world. Journal of Advanced Nursing 7(4): 327–336

Metcalf C 1987 Humour, life and death. Oncology Nurse Forum 14: 19–21

Mishminsky M 1991 Humour as a courage mechanism. Israelite Annual Psychiatry and Related Disciplines 15(4): 352–363

Parse R 1993 The experience of laughter: a phenomenological study. Nursing Science Quarterly 4: 69–75

Pasquali E 1990 Learning to laugh: humour and therapy. Journal of Psychosocial Nursing and Mental Health Services 28(3): 31–38

Pettifor J 1982 Practice wise: a touch of ethics and humour. Canadian Psychology 23(4): 261–263

Polit D, Hungler B 1985 Essentials of nursing. In: Polit D, Hungler B (eds) Research: methods, appraisal and utilization. J B Lippincott, Philadelphia

Robinson V 1977 Humour and the health professions. Charles B Slack, Thorafare, New Jersey

Rosenburg L 1989 A delicate dose of humour. Nursing Forum 24: 2

Rosenheim E, Golan G 1986 Patients' reactions to humorous interventions in psychotherapy. American Journal of Psychotherapy 40: 110–124

Royal College of Nursing 1977 Ethics related to nursing research. Royal College of Nursing, London

Schlesinter M, Yodfat Y 1988 Effect of psychosocial stress on natural killer cell activity. Cancer Detection and Prevention 12: 9–14

Schlinder L 1988 Understanding the immune system. Department of Health and Human Services, Washington DC

Scott C 1985 Go ahead, laugh, it's good for you. Nursing Success Today 2(1): 8

Siegel B 1986 Love, medicine and miracles. Harper and Row, New York

Simon J 1988a The therapeutic value of humour in ageing adults. Journal of Gerontological Nursing 14(1): 20–24

Simon J 1988b Humour techniques for oncology nurses. Oncology Nursing Forum 16(5): 667–670

Smith Lee B 1990 Humour relations for nurse managers . . . the positive and physiological and psychological benefits. Nursing Management 21(5): 80, 88–92

Sumners A 1990 Professional nurse attitudes towards humour. Journal of Advanced Nursing 15: 196–200

Vaillant G 1977 Adaptation to life. Cited in: Thorson J, Powell F 1993 Relationships of death, anxiety and sense of humour. Psychological Reports 72: 1364–1366

Warner S 1984 Humour and self-disclosure: within the milieu. Journal of Psychosocial Nursing and Mental Health Services 22(4): 17–21

Warner S 1991 Humour: a coping response for student nurses. Archives of Psychiatric Nursing 5(1): 10–16

Weisman A, Hackett T 1961 Predilection to death and dying as a psychiatric problem. Psychosomatic Medicine 23: 232

Wheaton B 1983 Stress, personal coping resources and psychiatric symptoms: an investigation of interactive models. Journal of Health and Social Behaviour 24: 208–229

Winnick C 1979 Cited in: Warner S 1991 Humour: a coping response for student nurses. Archives of Psychiatric Nursing 5(1): 10–16

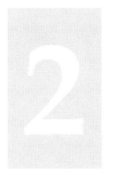

Skin-to-skin contact for premature and sick infants and their mothers

Kim Smith

Commentary

Nursing and midwifery knowledge is beginning to enter an exciting new phase. Conventional wisdom, that was often no more than pseudo-scientific moralizing, is being substituted by nursing and midwifery science. Increasingly, students challenge received wisdom and expect answers to profound problems. We do not always have those answers.

One way forward is to encourage local, small scale evaluations of practice – to identify the effectiveness of practices and to identify patient outcomes.

This study fits into that growing literature and makes a useful contribution to both evaluation and methodology. More such studies are needed and then we can aggregate these cases into a larger review, to chart the way towards evidence-based care.

This study is an excellent example of undergraduate research. Using a carefully designed methodology that incorporated physiological measurements and qualitative data collection techniques, Kim Smith has, as the title tells us, explored the effects of 'kangaroo-care' or the skin-to-skin contact of mothers and their premature and sick infants.

Kim describes a scenario where neonates were once nursed in an environment where only minimal handling was encouraged. This has changed in recent years and there has been the cautious development of a 'touching' or gentle contact ethos, perhaps typified by kangaroo-care, where infants are placed in direct skin-to-skin contact with their mothers. Kim performed a useful exploration of the relevant literature on the subject of touch, particularly related to neonates. As a result, she identified the need for further research in this area and formulated a hypothesis that kangaroo-care did not have an adverse effect on infants' physiological status. Using measurements of physiological parameters Kim found that this was indeed the case, that there were no adverse reactions. Indeed, it was found to have positive physiological benefits. In addition, mothers also reacted very positively to kangaroo-care.

Because of the small sample sizes, it would be unwise to generalize from the results of this carefully designed study. However, it does show that the potential benefits of kangaroo-care should be taken seriously, and it also shows that even small studies can be incredibly productive and significant. Perhaps somebody reading this chapter might like to replicate this research, leading to increased empirical support for what appears to be such a simple, yet effective, cost neutral intervention.

ABSTRACT

This study assessed the physiological effect of 'kangaroo-care' on 10 sick and premature infants being nursed on a neonatal intensive care unit (NICU), by using an open observational study. Secondly, it evaluated the psychological effect on the mothers who performed this care. Kangaroo-care involved skin-to-skin contact between a mother and infant by positioning the infant in an upright position between the mother's breasts. One hour before and after the kangaroo-care, the following observations of the infant were recorded: heart rate, respiratory rate, inspiratory oxygen requirements, oxygen saturation, sleep state and level of activity. The infant's axilla temperature was also recorded immediately before and after the kangaroo-care. During the hour before and after kangaroo-care the infant was nursed undisturbed in an incubator/cot. Parental reaction to the intervention was evaluated by the completion of a comment sheet.

The results indicated that the infants' physiological parameters were stable and in many cases improved during kangaroo-care. Temperature recordings were higher after kangaroo-care than before the intervention. Of the infants who had an oxygen requirement, there appeared to be a consistent reduction in inspired oxygen concentration during kangaroo-care. Heart and respiratory rate were also noted to be more stable during kangaroo-care. The experience was evaluated favourably by all parents involved. In conclusion kangaroo-care does not appear to have a detrimental effect on the physiological status of infants who are considered well enough to be taken out of an incubator or cot for a cuddle. It would also appear to provide parents with a psychologically rewarding alternative to the traditional cuddle.

INTRODUCTION

This work sets out to examine the effect of a relatively new intervention known as 'kangaroo-care' on the physiological status of 10 sick and premature infants and then evaluate the psychological responses of the mothers involved in this form of care.

Kangaroo-care involves skin-to-skin contact between a mother and her infant who, dressed only in a nappy, is placed in an upright position between the mother's breasts. Although technically a form of handling, kangaroo-care would appear to be no more physiologically stressful for the infant than being given a traditional cuddle or being nursed undisturbed in an incubator or cot (Affonso 1989, Anderson 1989, Leeuw 1991, Wahlberg 1992, Whitelaw & Sleath 1985). The whole ethos of kangaroo-care is centred around the infant and parent or caregiver, ensuring that the infant has the minimum of disturbance whilst being in a safe and nurturing environment. This ethos could be compared to that held in neonatal nursing prior to the mid-1950s. Until this period there was a widely held but poorly defined theory that preterm infants at the highest risk of mortality exhibited signs of 'congenital feebleness' (Budin 1907). This theory formed the basis of the care sick neonates received. These 'congenitally feeble' infants were protected from any disturbance nursing staff felt to be unnecessary; this even extended to actively discouraging doctors from fully examining infants (Silverman 1987).

The 1950s saw a complete change in the ethos of neonatal care, with a 'hands on' policy of clinical investigations and active treatment with drugs and physical agents. When this change in neonatal medicine began it was difficult to convince nurses who had spent years adhering to the 'hands-off' approach that the advantages of the new 'hands-on' approach would far outweigh any adverse effects it may have. With time, as infant mortality rates reduced and smaller infants survived, the initial anxieties of caregivers were reduced and the frequency and duration of handling these infants received increased (Silverman 1987).

However, in recent years concerns regarding the type, duration and frequency of handling that sick and premature infants are exposed to have resurfaced (Harrison et al 1990, Horsley 1988, Mok 1991, Tucker-Catlett & Holditch-Davis 1990, Weibley 1989). During this same period there has also been mounting conflicting research that demonstrates the importance of touch in the fragile parent–infant bonding process (Cusson & Lee 1994, Klaus & Kennell 1982, Rode 1981, Vietze 1990). This presents those caring for sick and premature infants with a dichotomy, resulting in a return to what Silverman (1987) called the 'hands on, hands off dilemma'.

In an attempt to resolve this 'dilemma' a distinction was sought between those types of handling episodes that may result in a negative effect on the infant's physiological status and those which may be expected to have a positive effect. When considering which types of interaction may provoke a deterioration in an infant's physiological status one might assume that non-interactional or procedural handling episodes would fall into the category of 'negative' touch, whilst interactional or parental handling could conversely fall into the category of 'positive' touch. However, research findings suggest that parental or interactional touch can potentially be as detrimental to the infant's physiological status as non-interactional or procedural touch (Horsley 1988, Korones 1976, Lawton & Melzer 1988).

The above therefore supports the premise of minimal handling for these sick and premature infants, but what of the parent's need to touch their baby and research that recommends maximum intervention and contact between infant and parent for the promotion of the bonding process? It is precisely this dichotomy that resulted in the search for a form of handling that would provide parents with a satisfying and pleasurable alternative to the traditional cuddle without physiological compromise to their infant's condition. Kangaroo-care appeared to be the panacea that was being sought.

LITERATURE REVIEW

TOUCH

Before the area of handling is considered the author feels it would be beneficial to use a conceptual framework to analyse the meaning of the term 'touch', allowing the differentiation of positive from negative touch at a latter juncture.

The following has been derived from the conceptual framework of Weiss (1979). Weiss purported that six factors constituted the language of touch: duration, frequency, location, intensity, sensation and action. The duration and frequency of handling, it was suggested, allows the body greater time for more pronounced physiological response. Location of stimulus contains two components: threshold, referring to the degree of innovation within the body area capable of response; and extent, the number of areas touched relative to the number of areas available to be touched. Intensity refers to the degree of indentation applied. Sensation refers to the immediate comfort or discomfort received from specialized receptors and transmitted to the brain. Finally, action refers to the rate of approach to a body surface.

This theory centred around the tenet that tactile interventions, if used appropriately, would result in facilitating an adaptation response in an individual. Conversely, if used inappropriately, it could result in the fostering of maladaptation behaviour (Weiss 1979).

With this conceptual framework in mind, an overview of the type of handling experiences infants being nursed in NICUs are exposed to would seem appropriate. This, it is hoped, will separate handling experiences that result in adaptation or improvement in physiological status from those resulting in maladaptation or a deterioration in physiological status. For this purpose infant handling experiences have been divided into:

1. *non-interactional or procedural touch*, defined by the author as uncomfortable or painful touch, which is usually associated with excessive handling or nursing/medical interventions.
2. *interactional touch*, defined by the author as a more gentle or soothing touch for the purpose of comforting or interacting.

Non-interactional touch

Despite an extensive literature search there appears to be very little research exploring the effect of non-interactional or procedural touch, as defined above, on the neonate. The majority of work into the behavioural or physiological changes in the neonate relate specifically to the response of the neonate to pain. Whilst it is acknowledged that the areas of pain and touch are undoubtedly interrelated, literature relating to the neonate's response to pain is not the key focus of this piece of work, therefore it will not be discussed directly but incorporated under other subject headings.

Thermoregulation

The thermoneutral environment is a narrow window of ambient temperature that produces the minimum of metabolic stress and oxygen demand on an individual (Merenstein 1993). This window of ambient temperature varies with an infant's age, body weight and clothing (Sauer 1984). A mechanically maintained thermoneutral environment, with the provisions of incubators and overhead heaters, is vital to the maintenance of the infant's status quo. Nursing and medical interventions or procedural touch all too often necessitate a disturbance in this environment, resulting in a reduction in the infant's temperature.

Mok et al (1991) studied the temperature changes associated with total nursing care procedures in 25 premature infants at 1 week of age. The birth weights of these infants ranged from 510 to 1500 g (median 920 g). The temperature changes from a total of 249 care procedures revealed a large drop in both central and peripheral temperature, with widening of the central peripheral temperature gap. The central temperature fell between 0.0 and 1.7°C (mean 1.7°C) and the peripheral temperature fell between 0.2 and 3.0°C (mean 1.3°C).

In full-term infants, a reduction in basal temperature leads to an increase in the metabolic rate and therefore oxygen demand, as the infant attempts to generate heat to regain a normal body temperature (Bell et al 1980). In premature infants with respiratory problems handling of any form, especially that of a non-interactional nature, as described by Mok (1991), may result in an increased oxygen demand in a neonate whose oxygen requirements may already be raised.

Oxygen requirements

A study by Glass (1968) into the physiological effect of procedural touch on the oxygen requirements of the neonate observed that in premature infants with respiratory problems, excessive handling often resulted in hypoxic episodes. This oxygen deficit resulted in an increased metabolic rate causing acidosis, hypoglycaemia and poor weight gain. The results of this work are supported by the findings of Speidel (1978), Long (1980), Norris (1981) and Beaver (1987), all of whom correlated excessive handling with an increased incidence of hypoxia in premature infants.

Norris et al (1981), in a study on premature and sick infants, found significant decreases in their oxygen saturation levels after endotracheal suctioning, repositioning and blood tests. These oxygen desaturations in 25% of the infants studied took in excess of 9 minutes to return to a baseline within acceptable parameters.

Peri/intraventricular haemorrhage

Peri/intraventricular haemorrhage (PIVH) is a frequently occurring problem that is a major determinant of the developmental outcome of the preterm infant (Merenstein 1993). The pathogenesis of PIVH is believed to be related to alterations in the cerebral blood flow that interacts with the immature brain to produce ruptures of the fragile capillaries in the germinal matrix (Merenstein 1993). While infants sustaining small germinal matrix haemorrhages may show no immediate or long-term effects, larger intraventricular or parenchymal lesions can result in varying degrees of motor and/or intellectual handicap, posthaemorrhagic hydro-cephalus or death (Graziani 1986, Roberton 1991). Currently, between 35 and 45% of all infants born prior to 35 weeks gestation are affected by the neurological deficits associated with PIVH (Volpe 1993).

The increased incidence of PIVH has been associated with procedural handling. One of the recommendations of a piece of research conducted by Kling (1988) was that in order to reduce the incidence of PIVH, nursing staff should critically evaluate all handling premature infants receive. Lawhorn (1988) describes a reduction in the incidence of PIVH following a change in NICU routines that were designed to provide individualized, develop-mentally supportive care, changes in the procedural handling of these infants being one of the major changes implemented.

Interactional touch

If, as the research above suggests, procedural touch elicits a 'nega-tive' physiological response from the infant one might surmise that parental or interactional touch would fall into the category of 'positive' touch, the soothing touch of the mother invariably being seen as the panacea to her infant's ills, but surprisingly this is not necessarily the case.

A study by Harrison et al (1990) evaluated the effect of parental touch on the heart rate and arterial oxygen saturation levels of 36 premature infants. The gestational age of the infants studied ranged from 27 to 33 weeks gestation at birth, the mean age being 29.6 weeks. The mean birth weight was 1337 g. In the 36 infants studied, there was no evidence of any obvious congenital abnormality and none had undergone surgery. The infants were videotaped during their parents' visits on up to three separate occasions during the infant's first month of life. Data on the infants' heart rate and oxygen saturation levels were recorded every 6 seconds. Physiological parameters were recorded three times on each of the three visits: before, during and after the parents' interaction with their baby. The results showed that the oxygen saturation levels during parental touch were lower than baseline on 45% and higher on 19% of visits. It was also found that oxygen saturation variability was greater during periods of parental touch and there were more abnormal oxygen saturation values during parental touch than during baseline periods. From this Harrison et al (1990) surmised that infants do respond physiologically to parental or interactional touch, but that indi-vidual responses may vary, with the response not always being favourable. There were decreases in mean heart rate during parent touch compared to baseline on 17% of visits, though none of the differences were clinically significant.

Gorski et al (1983) suggested that because acutely ill premature babies are so sensitive to stimulation, they respond as negatively to interactional touch as they do to procedural touch.

FREQUENCY OF INFANT HANDLING ON NICUs

Horsley (1988) studied the frequency with which infants in NICUs were handled. Eight infants were studied, their gestational ages ranged from 28 to 33 weeks, their ages from newborn to 17 days and their conditions ranged from an infant with mild respiratory distress who was being nursed in air to three infants who required mechanical ventilation. The time of the handling, the duration of the handling episode and the procedure or reason for handling were documented.

The results indicated that the mean number of handling episodes per 24-hour period was 47 times, ranging from 33 to 61 occasions. For the three ventilated infants the mean number of handling episodes over the same period was 55 times. This was considerably higher than that experienced by the unventilated infants whose mean number of handling experiences over the same period was 42 times. The study revealed the neonatal nurse to be the main perpetrator of this disturbance, handling the babies more frequently than the doctors on a ratio of 37:8. Conversely, parents handled their infants on average twice over a 24-hour period.

The infants involved in the study were also found to be handled at some point every hour. Between 0800 and 2400 hours the infants were recorded to have been handled between nine and 30 times an hour, this excessive handling obviously having a profound effect on the well-being of the infant. In a similar study premature infants were found to be disturbed on average 132 times a day, with undisturbed rest periods ranging from only 4.2 to 9.2 minutes (Korones 1976). Lawton & Melzer (1988) calculated that premature infants are handled for approximately 20% of the day.

The relentless handling that premature and sick infants being nursed on NICUs are exposed to, as discussed above, has a profound effect on the infants' immediate physiological status but current research suggests it may also have a more prolonged effect on the overall well-being of the infants by disrupting and depriving them of sleep.

SLEEP – A PHYSIOLOGICAL NEED

Preterm or sick neonates, like any newborn infant, if left un-disturbed will spend the majority of their day asleep. Unlike healthy newborn infants, sick neonates whose condition necess-itates admission to a NICU are, it would seem, handled constantly throughout the day and night (Horsley 1988, Korones 1976, Lawton & Melzer 1988). This constant handling will inevitably result in a disruption of sleep. Considering the premise that sleep is a basic physiological need (Maslow 1970), it would appear appropriate to review the literature pertaining to the effect of sleep deprivation on the neonate.

Premature infants have been found to fall asleep in active sleep and then complete sleep cycles consisting of both active and quiet sleep which last for 55–90 minutes, taking approximately 30 minutes to reach quiet sleep after falling asleep (Anders & Keener 1985, Watt & Strongman 1985). Quiet sleep is the most important and therapeutic of the sleep states, total relaxation bringing about a reduction in heart rate, respiratory rate and oxygen requirements (Watt & Strongman 1985).

Infants often change sleeping and waking states in response to environmental stimulation, nursing and medical intervention being a major cause of this stimulation. Blackburn (1982) claimed that due to procedural intervention infants on NICUs spend approximately 20 minutes a day in deep sleep and are therefore sleep deprived. It is this continuous arbitrary disruption of sleep patterns, resulting in a reduction of quiet sleep, that Adam & Oswald (1984) claimed is especially harmful for the acutely ill infant, as this sleep state is hypothesized to be necessary for healing.

PARENT–INFANT ATTACHMENT

The subject of parent–infant attachment or bonding has been open to considerable experimental investigation (Ross 1980, Seashore 1981, Sluckin 1983). However, it was Klaus & Kennell (1976) who first used the terms 'attachment' and 'bonding' to describe the process of relating between parent and infant. Klaus & Kennell, in the same work, also described a 'sensitive period' of time, initiated by the infant's birth and persisting for a number of days, during which a mother is particularly open to forming a relationship with her baby. It was suggested by the two authors that with the birth of a healthy infant this 'sensitive period' of parental attachment is assisted by simple acts such as touching, holding and caring for one's infant. Sucklin et al (1983), however, suggest that there is neither theoretical or empirical evidence to support the existence of a time-limited sensitive period.

The circumstances necessitating a premature or sick infant being nursed on a NICU inevitably result in an enforced separation of parent and infant. Separation has been purported to result in a disturbance of the parent–infant relationship by delaying or in some cases preventing attachment (Affonso 1989, 1992, Harmon 1981, Kaplan & Mason 1960, Klaus & Kennell 1976, 1982, Pederson 1987, Perehudoff 1990, Sugarman 1977, Trause & Kramer 1983, Zeanach et al 1984). The results of studies by Svejda (1980) and Rode (1981) failed to find differences in parent–infant attachment between groups where varying amounts of separation had occurred. Roberton (1992) suggests that neonatal events inevitably affect parent–infant attachment but that parent–infant relationships can develop after early separation.

KANGAROO-CARE

Kangaroo-care is a simple intervention that enables skin-to-skin contact between a parent and their infant. It has been so named as the infant is placed in a vertical position between the mother's breasts or on the father's chest, which resembles the method marsupials such as kangaroos use to care for their young (Anderson 1989).

This method of caring for premature infants was first introduced by physicians Dr Edgar Rey and Dr Hector Martinez (1979) of the Maternal Child Institute in Bogotá, Colombia. It was developed originally as an alternative to hospital care when a lack of incubators for single occupancy increased infection rates among premature infants. The Colombian mothers served as 'human incubators' for their premature infants, who survived in spite of their impoverished home confinements. It was felt that many of these infants would have died if the kangaroo method of care had not been implemented (Whitelaw & Sleath 1985).

Infants' response

A study by Luddington-Hoe (1990) was designed to test the efficiency of kangaroo-care for transitional care premature infants. The researchers addressed three clinical concerns: firstly, would the infant respond to kangaroo-care without physical compromise to heart rate, respiratory rate, oxygen saturation, percentage of quiet time characterized by periodic breathing and without apnoea or bradycardia? Secondly, would skin exposure during kangaroo-care contribute to body heat loss in preterm infants as measured by abdominal skin temperature? Finally, would there be any benefit to the infant in terms of sleep patterns? The findings of this research indicated that kangaroo-care had no adverse effect on the physiological variables measured. The infants were found to have more regular and even respirations and improved sleep patterns. The researchers concluded that healthy transitional care infants can tolerate 2–3 hours of kangaroo-care without cardiorespiratory or thermal compromise.

Affonso (1989) evaluated the effect of kangaroo-care on the physiological status of premature infants in an American NICU and found there to be no difference in the frequency or duration of apnoea, bradycardia, heart rate or oxygen saturation during skin-to-skin contact compared with those same variables taken before such contact. However, the percentage of sleep time and skin temperature of these infants were lower after the kangaroo-care than before. De Leeuw et al (1991) reported similar findings regarding stability of physiological parameters in low birth weight infants during kangaroo-care. It was suggested that kangaroo-care could have psychological benefits to the mother in terms of bonding and to infants purely as an alternative to being in an incubator or cot.

Luddington-Hoe (1990) studied energy conservation during skin-to-skin contact between premature infants and their mothers. This was evaluated by examining the effect of kangaroo-care on three indexes of energy expenditure: heart rate, activity level and behavioural state. The findings suggested that skin-to-skin contact results in a reduction in the energy expenditure of those infants involved. A similar study concerned with skin-to-skin contact and the growth patterns of low birth weight infants was undertaken by Schmidt (1986). This randomized controlled trial consisted of 23 premature infants, 12 of whom received kangaroo-care while the remaining 11 received standard care. The results indicated that there was an increase in the average weight gain, length and head circumference of the kangaroo-care infants.

Although the above studies have reported several benefits associated with kangaroo-care, interpretation and generalization of their findings are limited in many cases due to the small sample size, absence of quantification and also design limitations including absence of control groups.

Sloan et al (1994) attempted to rectify the shortcomings associated with some of the abovementioned research. This longitudinal, randomized, controlled trial undertaken in Quito, Ecuador, set out to compare the effects of kangaroo-care and standard treatment on morbidity, growth and cost of care for infants weighing less than 2000 g at birth. The participating infants were assigned by simple randomization to a kangaroo-care group or the standard treatment group. The infants were followed up until 6 months of age. The results of the study suggested that there were substantially lower incidences of severe illnesses, especially lower respiratory tract infections, in the kangaroo-care group. Kangaroo-care did not reduce neonatal mortality; as had been expected, most of the mortality occurred prior to the infants being recruited into the study. There was found to be no statistical difference in costs between the two groups.

While some studies purport kangaroo-care to have a significantly beneficial effect on the physiological status of the infant, other studies refute this and cite evidence suggesting the intervention has no significant effect on the infants' well-being. However, there has been no research to date that suggests kangaroo-care has a detrimental effect on the infants' physiological status.

Parental response

Much of the research pertaining to kangaroo-care is of a qualitative nature, relating to the psychological impact of undertaking this procedure on the mother. As with the studies into the physiological effect of kangaroo-care on the infant, no adverse reactions have been documented in the literature to date.

Affonso (1989) explored the effects of the kangaroo-care and standard neonatal care on maternal reaction. Sixty-six mother–infant pairs were recruited into the study. The total sample group was divided into two groups of 33 infants. The infants in one group received kangaroo-care while the infants in the remaining group received standard prematurity care. The results indicated that the mothers in the kangaroo-care group expressed confidence in breastfeeding, felt more comfortable in the NICU environment, visited their infant for long periods of time and expressed eagerness at the prospect of taking their infant home. These findings differed significantly from those received from the standard prematurity care group. These mothers experienced problems with their breastfeeding, felt uncomfortable in the NICU environment and were observed to be less frequent visitors to their infant. Affonso (1989) purported that skin-to-skin contact provided by kangaroo-care had eased the maternal pain and emotional suffering incurred by the multiple losses inherent in the birth of a premature infant. Schmidt (1986) highlighted the psychological gains found with mothers who undertook kangaroo-care. These included increased visitation, more frequent handling in the form of kangaroo-care and a greater capacity to communicate positive and negative emotions towards the infant than among mothers who had not undertaken kangaroo-care.

A considerably smaller study undertaken by Drosten-Brooks (1993) investigated the effect of kangaroo-care on the maternal caregiver. The results indicated that the initially nervous mothers soon became more confident in their abilities as a caregiver. However, the major recommendation of this piece of work was that NICUs need to be redesigned to allow parents privacy when carrying out interventions such as kangaroo-care.

Hamlin & Ramachandran (1993) described the reaction of parents of premature infants to kangaroo-care. Parents were described as having an '. . . indescribable feeling of joy' (p 16) due, according to the author of the study, to the fact that parents felt they were finally doing something for their infant.

Bosque (1988) set out to determine if kangaroo-care was a safe, feasible and beneficial method of caring for very low birth weight infants. Six infant–parent pairs were studied. The results indicated that heart rate, respiratory rate, incidence of apnoeas and oxygen saturations were similar in both groups. All mothers felt that the close and prolonged skin-to-skin contact provided by the kangaroo-care was beneficial to their relationship with their infant.

A study by Whitelaw et al (1988) investigated the maternal response to the introduction of kangaroo-care on a regional NICU. This study, in contrast to those above, did not observe significantly prolonged visiting times. However, each of the mothers involved in the study commented on the pleasure they derived from the kangaroo-care experience.

Skin-to-skin contact between mother and infant has also been documented as prolonging lactation in breastfeeding women. Whitelaw et al (1988) in a comparative study found that 55% of mothers in the kangaroo-care group lactated for more than 6 weeks, as compared to 28% of the non skin-to-skin handling group. These results compare favourably with Hamlin & Ramachandran (1993) who claimed that breastfeeding mothers who undertook kangaroo-care often experienced the physiological milk 'let-down' during the care. It was purported by Hamlin & Ramachandran (1993) that this encouraged mothers to continue expressing breast milk, promoted early breastfeeding and enhanced the breast-feeding success rate of the NICU. Several other studies into kangaroo-care have highlighted the increased incidence of sustained breastfeeding among women who regularly carry out the intervention (Affonso 1989, Armstrong 1987, Bosque 1988, Wahlberg 1992).

THE STUDY

AIM

The aim of the study was twofold: firstly to discover the physiological effect of kangaroo-care on premature and sick neonates and secondly to evaluate the feelings of the parents involved in this type of care.

The hypothesis was that kangaroo-care does not have a detrimental effect on the physiological status of premature and sick infants who are deemed well enough to be taken out of their incubator for a cuddle.

RATIONALE

Admission of a baby onto a NICU inevitably results in a disruption to the psychological bonding process between parent and infant (Klaus & Kennell 1982). Parents are encouraged to handle their infant in an attempt to 'normalize' this period of hospitalization and promote parent–infant interaction. Research has demonstrated that even parental touch can have a negative effect on the physiological status of the infant (Harrison et al 1990). Therefore an alternative form of handling technique has been sought. Kangaroo-care appears to provide parents with the opportunity for skin-to-skin contact with their infant without compromise to the neonate's physiological status (Affonso 1989, Luddington-Hoe 1990, Whitelaw & Sleath 1985).

ETHICAL CONSIDERATIONS

Ethical permission including verbal consent was initially sought by meeting with the two consultant neonatologists and the clinical nurse manager of the neonatal unit upon which the study was undertaken. During these meetings ethical considerations were discussed, resulting in all individuals giving their approval for the study to be undertaken.

Due to the nature of the research and the fact that it directly involved a client group, ethical approval was successfully sought from the ethics committee of the hospital group in which the study was to be undertaken.

Written consent was also sought from all parents whose infants were involved in the study.

DESIGN

To evaluate the effect of kangaroo-care on the physiological status of the infant a quantitative, open observational, descriptive design was employed. Conversely, a qualitative design was implemented to evaluate the retrospective feelings of the parents involved in the study. Polit & Hungler (1987) describe descriptive research as summarizing the status of the phenomenon as it currently exists. A design that described the characteristics of a group and identified relationships within that group was therefore considered an appropriately reliable framework from which the research question could be answered.

The following physiological observations were recorded from the infant:

1. Axilla temperature, measured using an electronic thermometer.
2. Heart rate, recorded from a cardiorespiratory monitor.
3. Respiratory rate, recorded from a cardiorespiratory monitor.
4. Oxygen requirements, measured from source if an oxygen requirement was present.
5. Oxygen saturation, recorded from a pulse oximeter from those infants whose oxygenation status required constant observation. The saturation monitor selected also displayed the infant's heart rate, thereby ensuring a correlation between the heart rate displayed on the cardiorespiratory monitor and the pulse oximeter and thus ensuring the accuracy of the oxygen saturation display.
6. Sleep state, assessed by observation. It was recorded whether the infant's eyes were open or closed and whether or not this was associated with behaviour that in the view of the observer represented a sleep state.
7. Activity level, assessed under one of two categories:
   - restless, being defined as generalized activity not thought to be associated with a sleep state;
   - settled, being defined as a quiet sleep state with the absence of any movement, with the exception of those movements considered by the observer to be associated with a sleep state.

The above physiological observations, with the exception of temperature, were recorded at 5-minute intervals for 1 hour prior to, during and after the kangaroo-care. The infant's axilla temperature was recorded on two occasions: immediately prior to the kangaroo-care, before the infant was taken out of the incubator/cot, and immediately upon the infant's return to the incubator/cot, after the kangaroo-care. All observations were recorded on a standard neonatal intensive care observation chart that had been adapted for the purpose of the study. During the 1-hour periods either side of the kangaroo-care the infant was left undisturbed and handling of the infant was only permitted if emergency intervention was necessary.

An evaluation of the maternal response to the kangaroo-care was sought upon completion of the intervention. This was achieved by requesting mothers to document their feelings, both positive and negative, relating to their kangaroo-care experience on a blank piece of A4 paper. Parents were encouraged to write both positive and negative comments, constructive criticism being actively encouraged.

PLACE

The research was undertaken on a 22-cot, medically orientated regional neonatal intensive care unit. Kangaroo-care had not been implemented on this unit prior to this study.

INCLUSION CRITERIA

The inclusion criteria permitted any premature or sick infant being nursed on the NICU whose physiological and neurological state had been deemed stable to be included in the study. Physiological and neurological stability were evaluated by the researcher together with the nurse caring for the infant and a member of the medical staff at senior house officer level or above. Physiological stability was evaluated as an assessment of:

1. temperature stability, defined for the purpose of this study as an axilla temperature between 36.5°C and 37.2°C with a good recovery after the infant had been handled;
2. absence of bradycardia or tachycardia, defined for the purpose of this study as a heart rate of less than 100 beats per minute or greater than 180 beats per minute respectively;
3. absence of apnoea, defined for the purpose of this study as any apnoeic episode within the previous 24 hours that necessitated cardiopulmonary resuscitation;

4. absence of oxygen desaturation with or without handling;
5. rapid recovery of baseline observations after procedures.

Neurological stability was assessed by an evaluation of the infants' generalized response to handling and the absence of fitting. Intraventricular haemorrhage (IVH) was discounted as a guideline to inclusion into the study as it was felt that even infants with relatively large cerebral bleeds are often physiologically stable and tolerate handling well. On the NICU where the study was undertaken, it was not policy to prevent infants being taken out of their incubator/cot purely on the basis of a significant IVH, unless the haemorrhage compromised the infant's condition in some way.

EXCLUSION CRITERIA

1. Infants deemed by the named nurse and a member of the medical team responsible for the infant's management, at senior house officer level or above, to be physiologically and/or neurologically unstable (see above).
2. Infants with a chest drain.
3. Infants with an umbilical, arterial or venous line.
4. Infants receiving vasopressors or non-depolarizing muscle relaxants.

RECRUITMENT

Parents whose infants were considered eligible for inclusion into the study were approached initially by the nurse caring for the infant. If the parents expressed an interest in becoming involved in the study an appointment was arranged at the parents' convenience for the researcher to meet with the parents on the neonatal unit. During this meeting a comprehensive explanation of the pertinent issues relating to the parents' and infants' involvement in the research was offered. Parents were also informed of the findings of comparable research that had examined the effect of kangaroo-care on the physiological status of sick and premature infants and the psychological effect on the caregiver. The following four points were also emphasized. Firstly, the researcher would be with the mother and her infant for the duration of the kangaroo-care. Secondly, if parents withheld their consent or conversely if consent was given and consequently withdrawn, it would in no way alter the care their infant received. Thirdly, if at any time during the kangaroo-care the parent wished to discontinue the intervention they were at liberty to do so and the kangaroo-care would be stopped immediately. Finally, if at any time during the kangaroo-care the infants exhibited signs of being distressed then again, the intervention would be stopped immediately. At the end of the meeting parents were provided with a written information sheet that reiterated the major points that were discussed. Persuasive tactics were not employed by the researcher in an attempt to encourage parents to recruit their infant into the study; conversely parents were actively advised to discuss their potential involvement and inform the researcher at a later juncture.

Verbal consent was also sought immediately prior to the kangaroo-care from the named nurse responsible for the care of the infant and a member of the medical team, at senior house officer level or above, as stated in the inclusion criteria.

THE SAMPLE

The original sample size for this study had aimed at recruiting 20 infants whose condition necessitated being nursed on a NICU and whose parents, due to the nature of their infant's condition, had limited physical contact with their baby. The amount and consistent nature of the data collected from the first 10 infants recruited into the study prompted the researcher to reconsider the sample size. It was decided to be appropriate to cease recruitment and concentrate on the analysis of the data obtained from a reduced sample size of 10.

The gestational age at birth of the recruited infants ranged from 26 to 41 weeks, the mean gestational age being 30.6 weeks.

The chronological age of the infants at the time of kangaroo-care ranged from 1 to 43 days, the mean chronological age being 17 days.

The actual weights of those infants involved ranged from 720 g to 2950 g, the mean weight being 1575 g.

The medical conditions of those infants involved ranged from a premature infant with surfactant-deficient respiratory distress syndrome requiring up to 75% oxygen therapy and ventilatory support to a premature infant with an infected vesicular rash being nursed in air.

The sample consisted of five infants with an oxygen requirement and five infants who were nursed in air. The recruitment of an equal number of oxygen-dependent and non-oxygen-dependent infants was a conscious decision by the researcher in an attempt to provide a valid representation of the infants being nursed on the NICU. The infants who required ventilatory support received this via continuous positive airways pressure (CPAP) ventilation. This provides a continuous positive end-expiratory pressure of an air/oxygen mix while not affecting self-initiated spontaneous respirations. This would therefore in no way affect the data collected regarding respiratory rate.

INTERVENTION

Mothers dressed in a front-opening garment were asked to position themselves comfortably in a rocking chair. Removal of bras was requested to improve skin-to-skin contact between the mother and infant and also to promote greater maternal comfort.

The infant, dressed only in a nappy, was transferred by the researcher to the mother, being placed in an upright position between the mother's breasts. Depending on the amount of equipment attached to the infant, a second nurse was occasionally required to assist with this procedure. A soft cotton sheet was then placed over the infant's body and secured laterally under the mother's arms. In addition, the mother's outer garments, in the case of a shirt or front-opening top, were also fastened around the infant's body. The back of the infant's head was sometimes

Table 2.1 Sample characteristics of study group prior to kangaroo-care

Subject number	M/F	Gestation at birth (weeks)	Birth weight (grams)	Age at KC (days)	Weight at KC (grams)	Condition at KC	Oxygen need (%)
1	M	26	920	19	940	Lung immaturity, ventilated	64–75
2	F	30	1640	6	1540	Lung immaturity, ventilated	68–78
3	M	32	2000	5	1830	Premature, nursed in air	21
4	F	32	1710	36	2660	Pulmonary atresia, nursed in air	21
5	F	26	800	19	720	Lung immaturity, ventilated	34–37
6	F	26	820	19	740	Lung immaturity, ventilated	25–28
7	F	27	1220	19	1260	Premature, nursed in air	21
8	M	28	1140	43	1360	Lung immaturity, ventilated	64–70
9	M	41	2950	1	2950	Birth asphyxia, nursed in air	21
10	M	38	1820	3	1750	Growth retarded, nursed in air	21

KC = kangaroo-care

Table 2.2 Characteristics of maternal study group

Subject	Age (years)	Gravida	Parity	Delivery: V/LSCS/Inst	Intended method of feeding (BF or AF)
1	28	1	1	V	BF
2	32	3	3	V	BF
3	35	2	1	V	BF
4	37	4	2	LSCS	BF
5	34	2	2	V	BF
6	34	2	2	V	BF
7	27	1	1	Inst	AF
8	30	4	1	LSCS	AF
9	26	3	2	V	BF
10	24	2	1	LSCS	BF

Key

Delivery
V – vaginal delivery
LSCS – lower segment caesarian section
Inst – instrumental delivery, e.g. forceps, Ventouse, etc.

Intended method of feeding
BF – breastfeeding
AF – artificial (bottle) feeding

covered for additional warmth. In the absence of this second layer of clothing an additional blanket was placed over the infant. Parents were encouraged to hold their infants for as long as they were comfortable or until the infant's condition necessitated being transferred back into the incubator.

The transfer of the infant back into the incubator or cot was achieved by loosening the outer garment or removing the blanket and then placing the infant, wrapped in the soft cotton sheet, back into the warmed incubator. Again, assistance was sometimes needed from a second nurse to help with the repositioning of equipment. Once in the incubator or cot, the infant's axilla temperature was recorded. To aid minimal disturbance upon the infant's return to the incubator, the soft cotton sheet was left covering the infant's body. Those infants returned to a cot were covered as before with the appropriate bedlinen.

MAINTENANCE OF CONFIDENTIALITY

Due to the nature of the research and the open-plan room dynamics of the intensive care nursery it was not felt necessary or practical to attempt to achieve confidentiality when carrying out the kangaroo-care. A screen was offered to all mothers that could be placed around the cot space to ensure a degree of privacy but in the experience of the researcher most mothers appeared to enjoy the attention they received from other parents and staff in the nursery.

Once the data had been collected confidentiality was maintained by allocating each infant and parent a number known only to the researcher that appeared on all documentation relating to the study.

The only individuals apart from the researcher who had access to the data collected as a result of the study were the clinical and academic supervisors of the research.

RESULTS

The results of both the quantitative and qualitative data are expressed in descriptive statistics. It was decided, upon discussion with the research supervisor, to concentrate the data analysis on the results obtained from the quantitative section of the study. The qualitative data therefore, although acknowledged as a significant contribution to the study, were analysed in less depth.

Ten mothers consented to themselves and their infants being involved in the study.

The time infants spent having kangaroo-care varied from 40 minutes to 1 hour, the mean duration being 48.6 minutes. Allowances were made in the calculations concerning the data obtained during the kangaroo-care sessions, thus ensuring that the data presented, although of varying lengths and therefore number of observations, were an accurate reflection of the information obtained.

All of the kangaroo-cares were ceased at maternal request, not due to a deterioration in any of the infants' physiological condition.

The following data analysis, relating to the physiological status

Table 2.3 Duration of kangaroo-care

Infant	Length of kangaroo-care (minutes)
1	45
2	60
3	50
4	60
5	50
6	60
7	55
8	40
9	60
10	60

Table 2.4 Axilla temperatures of infants before and after kangaroo-care, together with environmental setting and temperature pre intervention

Infant number	Temp 1 (°C)	Temp 2 (°C)	Environment at Temp 1	Environmental temp in incubator/cot (°C)
1	37.0	37.0	Incubator	33.0
2	37.1	37.2	Incubator	31.0
3	36.7	37.1	Cot	24.0
4	36.9	37.1	Cot	24.5
5	36.5	37.1	Incubator	32.0
6	36.8	37.0	Incubator	32.0
7	36.8	37.0	Cot	24.0
8	36.8	37.1	Incubator	32.5
9	36.5	37.2	Cot	25.0
10	36.7	37.1	Cot	24.0

of the infants during the study, will take place under the subject headings under which it was collected.

Temperature

The axilla temperature, in degrees centigrade (°C), of all 10 infants was recorded immediately before and after kangaroo-care. Table 2.4 gives an account of these data, with Temp 1 indicating the infants' temperature before the kangaroo-care and Temp 2 after kangaroo-care.

With the exception of Infant No. 1, whose temperature was static at both recordings, the remaining nine infants showed a consistent increase in axilla temperature after kangaroo-care.

The mean axilla temperature prior to kangaroo-care was 36.7°C and post kangaroo-care was 37.0°C (Fig. 2.1). A comparison of individual temperature increases post kangaroo-care resulted in a variation between 0.1°C and 0.7°C, giving a mean increase of

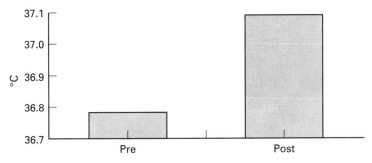

Figure 2.1 Axilla temperature pre and post kangaroo-care.

0.31°C. This result was interesting as five of the 10 infants were being nursed in an incubator, due in part to their inability to maintain their own body temperature in the ambient intensive care environment of 24–25°C.

Heart rate

The heart rate of all infants was measured at 5-minute intervals throughout the study. The heart rate of the neonate is expected to be between 110 and 160 beats per minute (Merenstein 1993).

In the hour prior to the kangaroo-care the mean heart rate of the study group was 164.5 beats per minute (bpm), the non-mean variation being 133–187 bpm and the difference between lowest and highest heart rate was 54 bpm.

During the kangaroo-care the mean heart rate was 150.8 bpm, the non-mean variation was 126–186 bpm and the difference between lowest and highest heart rate was 40 bpm.

Post kangaroo-care the mean heart rate was 154.3 bpm, the non-mean variation was 133–182 bpm and the difference between lowest and highest heart rate was 49 bpm (Fig. 2.2).

The mean heart rate post kangaroo-care (154.3 bpm) was higher than that recorded during the kangaroo-care (150.8 bpm) but not as high as that recorded prior to the intervention (164.5 bpm). The difference between lowest and highest heart rate was also slightly increased post kangaroo-care (49 bpm) in comparison to the difference during kangaroo-care (40 bpm), but again it is still lower than those observations recorded prior to the intervention (54 bpm).

The lowest heart rates, although still within acceptable limits, were recorded during kangaroo-care. As with adults, interventions

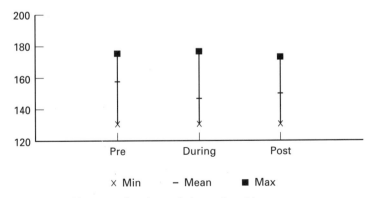

Figure 2.2 Heart rate (bpm) pre, during and post kangaroo-care.

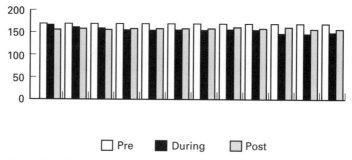

☐ Pre   ■ During   ☐ Post

Figure 2.3 Heart rate pre, during and post kangaroo-care. The x axis represents the 5-minute time intervals over which the information was recorded. The y axis represents heart rate (bpm).

that reduce the cardiac workload to the lower end of acceptable parameters are desirable (Roberton 1992).

The data also revealed irregular mean heart rates during the hour prior to the kangaroo-care. There was also no consistent trend in the mean heart rate during this period. However, during the kangaroo-care the mean heart rates consistently decreased from 163.7 bpm to 140.8 bpm at 55 minutes, with a slight increase to 142.8 bpm at 60 minutes. Post kangaroo-care, although no evidence of a continuation in this trend, there was less beat-to-beat variation in heart rate.

The above data and the emergence of certain trends are illustrated in Figure 2.3.

In summary the mean heart rate and heart rate range during kangaroo-care appeared, in general, to be lower than those recorded either prior to or after the intervention. However, although elevated post kangaroo-care, the mean heart rate and range were not as high as those recorded prior to the intervention.

All observations recorded were within acceptable limits.

Respiratory rate

The respiratory rate of all infants was measured at 5-minute intervals throughout the study. The respiratory rate of a neonate is expected to be between 20 and 50 breaths a minute (Merenstein 1993).

In the hour prior to the kangaroo-care the mean respiratory rate of the study group was 50.1 respirations per minute (rpm), with a non-mean variation of 22–85 rpm. The difference between highest and lowest respiratory rate was 63 rpm.

During the kangaroo-care the mean respiratory rate was 39.7 rpm, with a non-mean variation of 28–80 rpm. The difference between highest and lowest respiratory rate was 52 rpm.

After kangaroo-care the mean respiratory rate was 47.4 rpm, with a non-mean variation of 30–68 rpm. The difference between highest and lowest respiratory rate was significantly less, 38 rpm, than previously recorded.

There appeared to be a continuation in the aforementioned trend of an initially high mean followed by a reduction in the mean during the kangaroo-care and then a slightly increased mean postintervention, but not to a level as high as before kangaroo-care (Fig. 2.4). This trend was more apparent when a comparison of the study groups' mean individual respiratory rates pre, during and post kangaroo-care was made (Fig. 2.5). As with the heart rate, there is an obvious reduction in the respiratory rate in all 10 infants during kangaroo-care, as compared with that prior to the intervention. Similarly, upon return to the incubator or cot, for the first 10 minutes the trend of a reduction in respiratory rate appears to continue. This trend was then reversed 15 minutes after the kangaroo-care with an increase in respiratory rate. However, after an hour the respiratory rate is still less than that recorded prior to the kangaroo-care.

There also appeared to be another similarity in trends between that of heart and respiratory rate. The mean respiratory rates prior to the kangaroo-care appeared somewhat irregular, the non-mean difference between highest and lowest rate being some 63 rpm. However, over the course of the hour prior to the kangaroo-care, there was a reduction in the mean respiratory rate from the first recording of 51.2 rpm to the final recording of 49.9 rpm.

During kangaroo-care there emerged a significant trend of a reduction in respiratory rate, the mean respiratory rate at the commencement of the intervention being 46.5 rpm and at the end of the intervention being 35.0 rpm. The intervention also

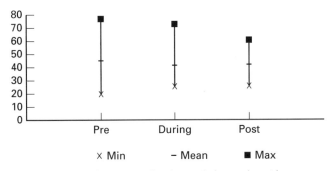

Figure 2.4 Respiratory rate (rpm) pre, during and post kangaroo-care.

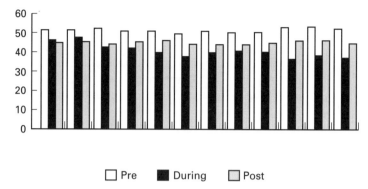

☐ Pre ■ During ☐ Post

Figure 2.5 Respiratory rate pre, during and post kangaroo-care. The x axis represents the 5-minute intervals over which the information was recorded. The y axis represents the respiratory rate (rpm).

appeared to have a slight stabilizing effect on the respiratory rate, the difference between highest and lowest respiratory rate being 52 rpm, but not significantly less than prior to kangaroo-care.

Post kangaroo-care presented the most significant reduction in the difference between highest and lowest respiratory rate with only a 38 rpm variation. Although the downward trend of respiratory rate seen during kangaroo-care was no longer present, the observations were generally more regular than those recorded prior to the kangaroo-care.

All observations recorded were within acceptable limits.

Oxygen requirements

Five of the infants in the study group had a generalized oxygen requirement in excess of 21% together with a need for continuous positive airways pressure ventilation. The remaining infants did not have an oxygen requirement greater than air. The study group for this analysis was therefore restricted to five infants. The infants' oxygen requirement was assessed against the oxygen saturation value and titrated accordingly.

The mean oxygen requirement prior to kangaroo-care was 55%, with a non-mean variation of 25–78%, the difference between lowest and highest oxygen requirement being 53%.

The mean oxygen requirement during kangaroo-care was 44.5%, with a non-mean variation of 21–78%, the difference between lowest and highest oxygen requirement being 57%.

The mean oxygen requirement post kangaroo-care was 47.7%, with a non-mean variation of 25–65%, the difference between lowest and highest oxygen requirement being 40% (Fig. 2.6).

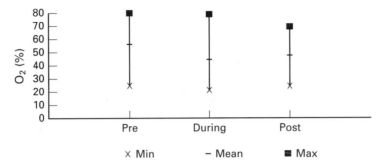

Figure 2.6   Oxygen requirements (%) pre, during and post kangaroo-care.

A comparison of the above three mean oxygen requirements revealed a continuation of the trend described during the analysis of heart and respiratory rate, the mean oxygen requirement being reduced by 9.5% from before the kangaroo-care to during the intervention. The post kangaroo-care mean oxygen requirement was 7.3% less than that recorded prior to the intervention (Fig. 2.7).

However, due to the reduced sample size for this analysis and the variation in oxygen requirement between individual infants, the mean oxygen requirement values were not felt to be representative of actual changes in oxygen requirements. The abovementioned trend is more apparent when each of the five individuals' oxygen requirement is viewed independently (Fig. 2.8).

Oxygen saturations

Infants requiring oxygen therapy are closely observed, by way of blood gas analysis and transcutaneous or saturation monitoring, to ensure they are receiving a therapeutic amount of oxygen. Oxygen saturation monitors record the percentage of red blood cells saturated with oxygen molecules. The upper and lower

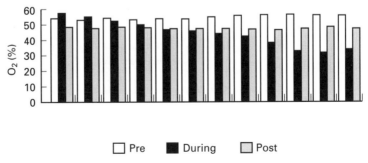

Figure 2.7   Oxygen requirement pre, during and post kangaroo-care.

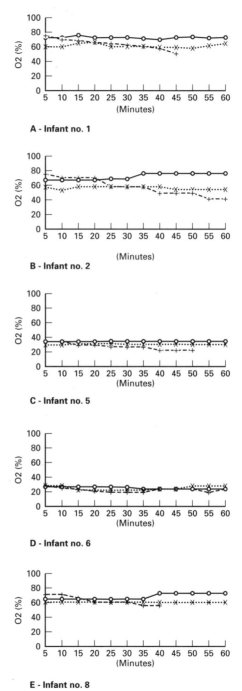

Figure 2.8   Individual oxygen requirements pre, during and post kangaroo-care for infants 1–5.

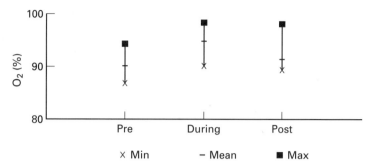

Figure 2.9 Arterial oxygen saturation pre, during and post kangaroo-care.

oxygen saturation parameters employed on the NICU where the study was carried out were 87% and 95%. For this reason, it was expected that there would be very little variation in oxygen requirements before, during and after kangaroo-care as it was the researcher's responsibility to titrate the oxygen supply according to the infants' requirements, ensuring that their saturations remained within the set parameters.

The oxygen saturation measurements were only recorded on the five infants with an oxygen requirement over and above that of air.

The mean oxygen saturation prior to kangaroo-care was 90.1%, with a non-mean variation from 86–94%, the difference between highest and lowest being 8%.

The mean oxygen saturation during the kangaroo-care was 93.8%, with a non-mean variation from 89–98%, the difference between highest and lowest being 9%.

The mean oxygen saturation post kangaroo-care was 91.1%, with a non-mean variation from 87–98%, the difference between highest and lowest being 11%.

The above data are illustrated in Figure 2.9.

It appeared that the mean oxygen saturation was marginally increased during the intervention but as was stated earlier, it was the responsibility of the researcher to ensure the infants' oxygen saturations were within the set parameters wherever possible. These data were included to support the validity of the previously documented data; the results of this section in themselves cannot therefore be considered as significant.

Sleep state

A scoring system was employed to indicate the sleep or wake state of the 10 infants throughout the study. The infants scored

1 if their eyes were closed and their overall appearance, in the opinion of the researcher, was interpreted as a sleep state. Conversely, a 0 was awarded for an awake state, defined as an alert state with open eyes.

Due, one would surmise, to the extremely rudimentary nature of the scoring system no significant conclusions could be drawn from the data obtained.

To assist with the interpretation of data, the total score of each infant in relation to their wake/sleep state was calculated and then converted into a percentage. Prior to kangaroo-care the study group were calculated to have spent approximately 32.5% of the hour in what was defined as an awake state. The remaining 67.5% of the hour was spent in a sleep state. The two states were not found to run concurrently one into the other; instead the pattern of sleep was found to be erratic. The minimum period of undisturbed sleep recorded was 5 minutes and the maximum length of sleep was 50 minutes. The mean duration of undisturbed sleep was 35 minutes.

During the intervention the study group were calculated to have spent 20.8% of the kangaroo-care in an awake state and 68.3% of the time in what was defined as a sleep state. The remaining 10.9% of the time accounts for unobtained data, as not all of the kangaroo-care episodes were of 60 minutes duration.

At the first 5-minute observation recording all 10 infants were found to have their eyes open. This awake state lasted for between 5 and 25 minutes, the mean duration being 10 minutes. Nine of the 10 infants studied were then observed to sleep for the remainder of the kangaroo-care, the tenth infant waking on one occasion at the end of the intervention for a period of 5 minutes.

The minimum period of this undisturbed sleep state was recorded at 30 minutes and the maximum duration was recorded at 55 minutes, thus giving a mean duration for undisturbed sleep as 40 minutes. The difference between the mean duration of undisturbed sleep prior to and during kangaroo-care was not felt to be representative of the actual difference observed in the raw data. This is thought to be due to the variation in duration of individual kangaroo-cares, hence a reduced amount of data was obtained during this period, whereas observations were recorded on all infants for a statutory 1 hour prior to the intervention. However, the difference in minimum duration of undisturbed sleep, 5 minutes pre kangaroo-care as compared to 30 minutes during the intervention, was felt to be significant.

Post kangaroo-care, the study group were calculated to have spent 18.4% of the hour with their eyes open in an awake state

Table 2.5 Summary of data pertaining to sleep state (n = 10)

	Prior to KC	During KC	Post KC
Total time asleep	67.5%	68.3%	81.6%
Total time awake	32.5%	20.8%	18.4%
Duration of undisturbed sleep:			
Minimum	5 min	30 min	5 min
Maximum	50 min	55 min	60 min
Mean	35 min	40 min	35 min

and 81.6% of the hour in a sleep state. The data suggest that the sleep obtained by the infant during this hour was of a slightly less settled nature than that observed during the kangaroo-care, the minimum duration of undisturbed sleep being 5 minutes and the maximum duration being 60 minutes. The mean duration of undisturbed sleep was 35 minutes (Table 2.5).

Level of activity

A similar scoring system to that utilized in the previous section was employed to indicate the level of activity exhibited by the infants. Infants were attributed a score of 1 if they appeared, in the opinion of the researcher, to be restless. Conversely, a 0 score was attributed to behaviour, or a level of activity, observed by the researcher to be of a settled nature.

Due again to the rudimentary nature of this scoring system, the data obtained resulted in a very limited interpretation.

To assist with the interpretation of data, as with the data obtained for sleep state, the total score of each infant in relation to their activity level was calculated and then converted into a percentage of the overall period. Prior to the kangaroo-care the study group were calculated to have spent approximately 26.6% of their time in what was defined as a restless state. The remaining 73.4% of the time was calculated to have been spent in a settled state. As expected, these results are comparable to those observations recorded on sleep state, prior to the intervention the infants spending 32.5% of the hour in an awake state and the remaining 67.5% of the time in a sleep state. Again, the periods of time spent in a settled state were variable, the minimum duration of a settled period being 5 minutes, the maximum period being 60 minutes. The mean period of settled behaviour was 27 minutes.

During the intervention the infants were calculated to have spent a significantly reduced period, 5.8% of the kangaroo-care, in a restless state. This was observed during the latter minutes of the kangaroo-care and appeared to be related to maternal movement. The maternal movement appeared to result from mild discomfort related to sitting in one position for up to an hour or as a result of preparing to transfer the infant back into the incubator/cot. The duration of time spent in a settled state was calculated at 83.3% of the intervention, the difference between the two values, 10.9%, resulting from the variation in duration of kangaroo-care. Differences occurred when a comparison of the data pertaining to sleep state prior to and during kangaroo-care was made. Prior to the intervention the data suggested that when awake, infants were generally in a restless state. However, during kangaroo-care infants were recorded to spend more time in a settled state when awake. During this settled awake period infants appeared to be actively looking around and attempting eye contact with their mothers. The other significant difference was the duration of settled periods during the intervention. The minimum period of individual continual settled behaviour was 15 minutes, the maximum period was 60 minutes. The mean period of continual settled behaviour for all 10 infants was 40 minutes, a significant increase on that observed prior to the kangaroo-care.

The observations recorded upon the infants' return to the incubator demonstrated a continuation of settled behaviour, with 85.9% of the hour being spent in such a state and the remaining 14.1% of the hour in unsettled behaviour. As expected, this period of restless behaviour appeared to be a direct result of the infant being returned to the incubator/cot. The duration of periods of settled behaviour remain very similar to those experienced during the intervention, the minimum period of continuously settled behaviour being 15 minutes and the maximum period being 60 minutes. The mean period of continuously settled behaviour was calculated at 35 minutes, only 5 minutes less than that recorded during kangaroo-care (Table 2.6).

Table 2.6 Summary of data pertaining to activity level (n = 10)

	Prior to KC	During KC	Post KC
Total time in settled state	73.4%	83.3%	85.9%
Total time in restless state	26.6%	5.8%	14.1%
Duration of settled behaviour:			
Minimum	5 min	15 min	15 min
Maximum	60 min	60 min	60 min
Mean	27 min	40 min	35 min

Maternal response

After they had carried out the kangaroo-care, mothers were requested to document their feelings, of both a positive and negative nature, on a blank piece of A4 paper. Ten completed comment sheets were returned, on either the day of the kangaroo-care or the day after the intervention had taken place. The researcher had anticipated brief responses to this request, but each returned comment sheet consisted of at least one completed side of A4 describing in detail some very emotive feelings. Despite the mothers having been encouraged to document any thoughts relating to their experience, no negative responses were submitted.

The following themes emerged from the returned comment sheets. Without exception, all 10 of the mothers commented on how difficult they had found the restricted contact that having an infant on a NICU inevitably brings. The mother of a 30-week gestation infant wrote:

One of the strongest feelings I have had since my baby was born is the urge to take her out of the incubator and hold her to me and cuddle and comfort her.

Another mother commented that:

I have felt that there has been little physical contact with my baby since his birth and have accepted this as necessary, but it was such a pleasure to hold him really close and give him a proper cuddle, feeling the warmth of him on my skin.

The feeling of skin-to-skin contact appeared to have an almost overwhelming effect on all of the mothers involved in the study. An observation made by the researcher during the kangaroo-care was that mothers who were usually very talkative became very quiet during the intervention; if they spoke at all it was in hushed tones to their infant. One mother was obviously aware of this and wrote:

For the first time since my little girl had been born I felt very very close to her . . . It was a beautiful feeling, even though I was in a room full of people I felt my baby and I were the only ones there.

Three of the mothers directly expressed a feeling of greater confidence when handling their infant. This appeared to be related to the satisfaction, in the mothers whose infants had an oxygen requirement, of observing a decrease in oxygen requirements associated with the intervention they were carrying out.

I just could not believe how his oxygen had to keep being turned down. By the time we'd finished the kangaroo-care he was in less oxygen than he'd ever been in. What made me feel really good was the thought that this was the first thing that I had been able to do to help my baby since he had been born. When I went home I cried!

A direct analogy was made by one mother of the similarity between the emotional feeling associated with breastfeeding her first child and those she experienced carrying out kangaroo-care:

It was nice to feel her warmth as she is too young as yet to breastfeed; it is the closest I have felt to breastfeeding and the bond that breastfeeding brings.

Similar comments relating to the effect of kangaroo-care on the breastmilk production of the mothers involved in the study also emerged. The mothers of premature or sick infants who are unable to breastfeed often experience a poor let-down response of breastmilk when using an electric breast pump. Of the 10 mothers involved in the study, eight intended to breastfeed and had been using such a device to express their breastmilk. Without exception, each of these eight mothers commented that on previous occasions the use of the breast pump had yielded a minimal milk supply, but that when they expressed their milk post kangaroo-care their milk production was significantly increased. The comment of one mother, who 4 days previously had decided to discontinue expressing breastmilk for her 43-day-old ventilated infant who was unable to breastfeed, was:

I used the breast pump every 6 hours during the day for 5 weeks and my milk supply went from very little to less. I tried everything to improve my milk supply but I was only getting off about 10 ml at a time, so I decided to stop expressing and put my baby onto formula milk as I just didn't think I had enough milk. Today I gave my baby a kangaroo cuddle for the first time. After my breasts felt very full, I went home and expressed off 70 ml in just 10 minutes.

Five of these breastfeeding mothers also commented on the fact that when they were carrying out the kangaroo-care they were aware of the physiological let-down reflex associated with breastfeeding. One mother commented that:

After a few minutes of the kangaroo-care she began to make sucking and rooting movements so I gave her my finger to suckle and some of my breastmilk started to leak out.

Interestingly, six of the 10 mothers commented in great detail upon the effect they perceived the kangaroo-care to have on their infant. One mother's account stated that:

After about 5 minutes we were both very relaxed. My baby started to go to sleep and her facial muscles got slacker and slacker, where her eyes had been quite 'screwed up' before, she relaxed and the skin smoothed right out. Throughout the kangaroo-care she hardly moved and her hands and body were quite 'heavy'. She lay very still and quiet, she was the most settled I had ever seen her.

The above analysis consisted of a generalized account of the maternal responses to kangaroo-care as opposed to an indepth individual analysis of each mother's response. However, several recurrent themes were identified:

1. improved physical contact between mother and infant;
2. feeling of psychological closeness between mother and infant;
3. increased maternal confidence;
4. increased breastmilk production;
5. affirmation that kangaroo-care was considered an acceptable and pleasurable alternative to a conventional cuddle.

DISCUSSION

INFANTS' RESPONSE
Axilla temperature

Core temperature readings are recognized as a more accurate evaluation of temperature, as they change only when maximum effort to preserve, produce or dissipate heat has failed (Darnall 1987). However, the arbitrary recording of rectal (core) temperatures was not in accordance with the policy of the NICU upon which the study was undertaken, therefore axilla (peripheral) temperature recordings were used.

Axilla temperatures for all infants were within normal range during all periods. The mean axilla temperature throughout the study was never less than 36.5°C, that recognized as resulting in minimal oxygen consumption in these infants (Buetow & Klein 1964).

One of the main concerns voiced prior to undertaking this study related to the low birth weight infants' ability to maintain their temperature if kept out of the incubator for extended periods of time. Three of the 10 infants, who had been nursed in a mean incubator temperature of 32°C, weighed between 720 and 940 g at the time of kangaroo-care. These infants, as with the others, were dressed only in a nappy during the kangaroo-care, with their mother's body heat, together with a soft sheet and the mother's outer clothing or blanket covering them, to maintain their temperature. However, as can be seen, no reduction in peripheral temperature was experienced by any of the infants during the intervention. The increase in peripheral temperature during kangaroo-care is therefore considered to be an important finding. Similar studies demonstrating maintenance of infant temperature during kangaroo-care have been cited in the literature (Acolet & Modi 1992, Luddington-Hoe 1990, Wahlberg 1987, Whitelaw et al 1988).

Several explanations are tentatively put forward to explain this increase in axilla temperature during kangaroo-care. The warm maternal skin, it could be suggested, may have reduced the infant's conductive heat loss, which commonly occurs as a result of being nursed next to or on a cold surface. The mother's warm skin in contact with one side of the infant's body, together with the outer clothing covering the other side of the infant, might also reduce convective (heat loss by moving air currents) and radiative (heat loss into large cooler environment) heat loss.

The researcher is aware that the maximum duration of kangaroo-care during this study was 60 minutes and although there was no reduction in any of the infants' axilla temperatures, careful monitoring of infants undergoing this intervention for increased time periods would be recommended.

Heart and respiratory rate

It was decided that the discussion and analysis of these results should be undertaken simultaneously due to the similarity in trends that occurred between the two observation parameters.

All observations relating to heart and respiratory rate were within normal limits during the study period.

In general, the transfer process of the infant from the incubator or cot appeared to be the least well-tolerated part of the skin-to-skin holding process. Although both the heart and respiratory rates remained lower than prior to the intervention there is little significant difference between the observations recorded within the first 10 minutes of kangaroo-care and those recorded prior to the intervention. After approximately 10–15 minutes of kangaroo-care the mean heart and respiratory rates began to decrease. A trend appeared in the cardiac and respiratory recordings of all 10 infants. The initially elevated recordings of both heart and respiratory rate in the hour prior to the intervention were followed by a gradual reduction in rate during kangaroo-care. The hour following the intervention saw a slight increase in these values but not to a level as high as those recorded prior to kangaroo-care.

It could be suggested that many of the qualities inherent in kangaroo-care may account for this reduction in the infants' heart and respiratory rates. Grimwade et al (1970) cite the familiar maternal voice and heart beat, heard as the infant lies against the mother's chest wall, as having a calming effect on the infant and therefore reducing cardiorespiratory rate. The sound of a heart beat has also been found to reduce crying and induce sleep in term newborn infants (Detterman 1978). The infants in the study group also experienced the movement of the mother's chest during respiration. Such movements, not routinely experienced by the infant nursed in an incubator or cot, have been claimed to pacify infants (Cunningham & Anisfield 1987, Korner et al 1983). The use of a rocking chair by the mothers during kangaroo-care was a conscious effort on the part of the researcher to provide an exaggeration of this rhythmical movement.

The mean heart and respiratory rates recorded upon the infants' return to the incubator or cot revealed an expected increase in these previously reduced observations. One can only assume that this physiological reaction of the infant resulted from being removed from the soothing environment next to the mother's warm skin and being placed in a less natural environment. What was unexpected was the fact that the heart and respiratory rates recorded on each of the 10 infants after the kangaroo-care, although increased, never became as high as those recorded prior to the intervention. It can only be surmised that, although not as settled upon their return to the incubator or cot, the infants were still physiologically benefiting from the kangaroo-care experience.

The reduction in heart and respiratory rates seen during kangaroo-care is an important clinical finding. Woodson et al (1983) claimed that the NICU environment can cause increases in cardiac and respiratory rates in acutely ill infants, resulting in increased oxygen consumption and calorific requirements. Luddington-Hoe (1990) suggested that a reduction in cardiopulmonary effort was directly related to a reduction in energy expenditure. It would seem, therefore, that a reduction in the infants' cardiac and respiratory rates to values at the lower end of acceptable parameters is of benefit to the physiological status of the infant. A reduction in these two observations has been associated with a reduction in stress in the infant (Grimwade et al 1970, Korner et al 1983). Much research has been undertaken that demonstrates the negative effect of the NICU environment on the infant (Gorski et al 1983, Horsley 1988, Norris 1981). An increase in the cardiopulmonary rate is frequently cited as an indicator of stress in the neonate (Bell et al 1980, Glass 1968, Lawhorn 1988, Long 1980, Mok 1991,

Speidel 1978). The reduction in heart and respiratory rates during kangaroo-care would therefore appear to assist in the reduction of the stress response in sick and preterm infants and was therefore to be considered a significant clinical finding.

Oxygen requirement and oxygen saturation

These two observations will be discussed together due to their integral nature.

Of the 10 infants in the study group, five had an oxygen requirement greater than air and required continuous positive airways pressure ventilation. The remaining infants were nursed in air, without need for mechanical ventilation. Oxygen requirement and saturation recordings were only carried out on those infants with an oxygen requirement greater than air.

The data pertaining to oxygen saturation levels were included to demonstrate that any changes in the infants' inspired oxygen concentrations occurred without detrimental effect to their oxygen saturation levels. An attempt was made to maintain their oxygen saturations between 87% and 95%.

The trend seen in the data relating to cardiac and respiratory observations was also apparent in the data relating to oxygen requirements. The transfer of the infant from the incubator or cot to the mother was reflected in a stasis of oxygen requirements. This 'transitional period' coincides with that evident in the cardiopulmonary results. The reluctance of the researcher to instigate major changes in oxygen requirements due to the effect of hyperoxia or hypoxia on the premature infant (Roberton 1992, Merenstein 1993), is reflected in the very gradual decline in inspiratory oxygen requirement. This also accounts for the plateauing of results over several minutes. Despite this, there was a significant reduction in mean oxygen requirements during the kangaroo-care from 57% to 35%.

Oxygen is a particularly dangerous therapy. Its use in the premature neonate is monitored intently as it is associated with retinopathy of prematurity and bronchopulmonary dysplasia (Roberton 1992, Merenstein 1993). Any intervention that results in a reduction in an infant's oxygen requirement is therefore a significant finding.

One could purport that the reduction in oxygen requirement occurred for similar reasons to those cited for the reduction in cardiorespiratory rate during kangaroo-care, that is, as a result of the infant feeling secure and content during the period of skin-to-skin contact with its mother. The reduction in energy expenditure due to a reduced cardiopulmonary rate has also been suggested as resulting in a decreased oxygen need (Luddington-Hoe 1990). One other additional factor may be the infant's upright position during kangaroo-care. A study by Picton-Warlow & Meyer (1970) suggested that pulmonary compromise was found when infants were nursed in side-lying positions, there being increased pulmonary function when infants are nursed in an upright position (as with kangaroo-care).

Behaviour and sleep state

These two observations will be discussed together due to the nature of the data obtained.

When considering how to assess the sleep state and activity level of the infants involved in the study, a very simplistic scoring system was decided upon. It was anticipated that the system used would provide enough data to present an overview of the infants' behaviour throughout the study. The author was aware of the lack of objectivity inherent in such a scoring system, but felt that the use of a more comprehensive system would be impractical. However, as was stated in the results section, the data were unexpectedly simplistic and therefore resulted in a limited interpretation of results.

During the hour prior to the kangaroo-care the observations indicated that the infants spent the majority of the time in a settled (73.4%) sleep (67.5%) state, the mean duration of this settled sleep state being 27 minutes and 35 minutes respectively. During this period it was noted that infants became restless almost immediately upon waking. No intervention was initiated by the researcher or the mother to pacify the infant during this period. The behaviour of all infants during this period was felt by their parents to be characteristic.

The data gained as a result of the observations recorded during this period were in stark contrast to those observed in the previous hour. The infants were all observed to be awake for up to 15 minutes after the commencement of the intervention. However, during this period the infants were generally observed to be content, actively looking around and in some cases attempting to achieve eye contact with their mother. This quiet alert state was unexpected and had previously never been observed by several of the mothers.

Upon the infants' return to their incubator/cot there was a generalized restless period among them, probably as a result of being removed from the comfort of their mothers. However, without exception, a settled sleep state was soon resumed by all infants.

When reviewing the literature in preparation for this study it was apparent that sick and premature infants require sleep and lengthy periods of settled behaviour in order to grow and improve their physiological status, awake states being cited as more costly, in terms of energy expenditure, than sleep states (Brooke 1979). Handling of infants is often considered synonymous with a disruption of this settled sleep state. The results of this study, although rudimentary, suggest that kangaroo-care provided the infants involved with an alternative, nurturing environment from which extended periods of settled sleep were obtained.

MATERNAL RESPONSE

All mothers evaluated the time they spent giving their infant kangaroo-care as a positive and personally beneficial experience. From the statements of the mothers five themes emerged. Firstly, all parents expressed approval of the increased physical contact implicit in kangaroo-care. The intimate nature of the skin-to-skin contact was also commented upon, if not directly on the comment sheet then to the researcher while carrying out kangaroo-care. Due to the strength of this particular response, it could be suggested that the skin-to-skin contact inherent in kangaroo-care may offer some parents an effective method of overcoming some of the barriers to attachment imposed by the infant's admission to a NICU.

During the preliminary conversation between the researcher and the mother regarding possible recruitment into the study, parents often asked for affirmation that the intervention would be ceased at their request if they so wished. This reassurance was always given and often repeated immediately prior to the kangaroo-care being carried out. In the event, each of the 10 parents was very reluctant to stop the kangaroo-care. It was observed by the researcher that during the kangaroo-care the confidence of the mothers in handling their infants increased. Once the mothers could see that the infants' physiological status did not deteriorate as a result of the kangaroo-care but remained stable and in many cases improved, their confidence improved. Mothers themselves commented on the personal satisfaction of knowing that it was their intervention in carrying out the kangaroo-care that had brought about the positive changes in their infants' physiological status.

Mothers were also aware of how settled their infants appeared during the kangaroo-care. This in itself was considered a worthy observation, as the mothers of premature infants spend the majority of their time simply looking at their infant. In the experience of the researcher, parents very quickly learn to interpret even the most subtle of behavioural cues from their infant. This awareness of their infants' relaxed state helped to compound those feelings mentioned above.

One of the most frequently reported comments was from the eight mothers in the study group who were intending to breast-feed their infants. Without exception, each of these mothers commented on their increased breastmilk supply upon expressing their milk after a kangaroo-care. Five of these mothers also commented that while carrying out the kangaroo-care they had experienced the physiological let-down response associated with breastfeeding. These are significant findings as mothers who wish to breastfeed their premature or sick infant often have to wait several weeks and in some cases months before the infant is mature or well enough to attempt a breastfeed. Previous studies, as documented in the literature review, have also commented on the association between kangaroo-care and improved lactation.

The hospitalization of a sick or premature infant, as illustrated in the literature review, often results in an interruption of the parent–infant attachment process (Affonso 1992, Harmon 1981, Klaus & Kennell 1982, Noble 1981, Sugarman 1977, Trause & Kramer 1983, Zeanach et al 1984). Parents are faced with continual barriers between themselves and their infant. Equipment, incubators and even research claiming that minimal handling will improve the infant's status quo all appear to conspire against the parent's vain attempts to form some sort of relationship with their infant. Although the ethos of minimal handling has never been in doubt, what has been questioned is the blanket statement that all handling episodes are detrimental to the well-being of the sick infant. It would appear from the results of this research that this is not so. The parent's psychological needs require equal consideration as the physiological needs of their infant. There is without doubt, in the experience of the author, an overwhelming parental urge to cast aside these 'barriers' in an attempt to initiate the attachment process. Touch is often the first step in achieving this. Kangaroo-care may help in facilitating this process. The results of this study suggest it to be a rewarding alternative to the 'conventional cuddle', the difference in the two being the closeness that the skin-to-skin contact provides the caregiver.

CLINICAL IMPLICATIONS

In Britain sick and premature infants are generally nursed in an incubator or cot, occasionally being taken out in order that their parents can give them a cuddle. Nurses are faced with the daily dichotomy of regular parental requests for increased interactional touch against the nursing and medical research that suggests the ill effects of all forms of touch on the sick or premature infant.

The author is extremely sympathetic to this dilemma. However, it is felt that the consistent nature of the results from the research carried out into kangaroo-care provide the nurse with a viable alternative form of handling experience to offer parents.

As with any intervention that directly involves the neonate, clinical judgement is recommended prior to considering the eligibility of an infant for this type of care. For the purpose of this study, strict exclusion criteria were exercised, ensuring that only those infants who were considered well enough to tolerate being taken out of their incubator were given kangaroo-care. The author, while recognizing the possible advantages of the intervention to both mother and infant, acknowledges that kangaroo-care is not suitable for all infants.

The results of the data pertaining to the effect of kangaroo-care on the physiological status of the infant are of clinical significance. In the experience of the author, one of the most frequently stated reasons why parents should not handle their infant is that of unstable temperature. In circumstances such as these, the parents sit watching their infant through the perspex incubator wall. The results of this study suggest that the study group's mean peripheral temperature actually rose during the intervention. This suggests a case for kangaroo-care in such circumstances.

The reduction and more regular cardiorespiratory rates seen during kangaroo-care present the nurse with an alternative form of positioning to be considered when planning the care of infants in the NICU. As was stated earlier, a reduction in pulmonary and cardiac workload, while still within acceptable parameters, is desirable in sick and premature neonates.

Kangaroo-care therefore has several nursing implications. Its limited use in this country, however, prevents larger scale research into further benefits.

LIMITATIONS OF THE STUDY
Literature review

Due to the recent introduction of kangaroo-care into the speciality of neonatal nursing (Rey & Martinez 1979), there are relatively few data documented in the literature. Of the research available, the sample sizes are limited and they present with methodological inaccuracies so may not be considered as statistically valid. However, the results of this type of intervention stand on their own, kangaroo-care being carried out as routine practice in many NICUs throughout the world.

The sample and sample size

The major criticism of the study was size. The researcher had initially intended to recruit 20 infants into the study. However, the results obtained by the time 10 infants had been recruited showed a similarity in trends within the data so it was therefore considered as a viable sample size, although recognizably small. The reduction in sample size allowed the researcher to undertake a qualitative analysis of the maternal response to the intervention. This had not originally been considered due to the time and word limitations of the study.

The researcher would have also liked to recruit some fathers into the study, but felt that by restricting the study group to mothers it would help avoid a possible extraneous variable.

The research instrument

The research tool was felt to be an appropriate method of collecting data. Concern was felt by the researcher regarding the rudimentary definitions employed to define wake/sleep states and activity level. At the commencement of the study this very basic scoring system was felt to be satisfactory. However, a more comprehensive scoring system that differentiated between various sleep states would be required in order to make any significant inferences relating to the infants' sleep state or activity level.

Analysis and interpretation of findings

The descriptive analysis was felt retrospectively to be restricted in its areas of observation. Either a more indepth analysis of fewer variables or the introduction of other physiological observations such as blood gas analysis may have been beneficial.

The researcher had at no point intended that the qualitative analysis would account for equal space within the study. It was, however, hoped that the results elicited from this would complement the results obtained from the quantitative data analysis. Due to the emotive nature of the maternal response to the kangaroo-care a more comprehensive analysis of the data would have been desirable.

Due to the intrinsically difficult nature of neonatal research much of the interpretation of the data was circumspect, there being very little research to support or refute the tentative suggestions that were put forward.

CONCLUSION AND SUMMARY

The hypothesis cited at the commencement of this study was that kangaroo-care does not have a detrimental effect on the physiological status of sick and premature infants who are deemed well enough to be taken out of their incubator for a cuddle.

The results of this study support the hypothesis, the following conclusions having been drawn from the data:

1. Thermoregulation was maintained during kangaroo-care even for infants of 720 g.
2. Cardiac and respiratory rates were reduced during the intervention, but remained within acceptable parameters.
3. There was a reduction in inspired oxygen concentration in those infants with an oxygen requirement.
4. The infants spent a greater period of time either awake and settled or asleep and settled than before or after kangaroo-care.

The study also set out to evaluate the maternal response to the kangaroo-care. Without exception, the maternal response to the intervention was favourable. Several themes emerged from the data:

1. Mothers enjoyed the physical contact and closeness inherent in kangaroo-care.
2. There was an increase in maternal confidence and satisfaction in being able to carry out the kangaroo-care.
3. An increase in breastmilk production was reported in all of the mothers who intended to breastfeed their infants.
4. Mothers also commented on how relaxed their infants appeared during kangaroo-care.

The results of this study suggest that kangaroo-care does not have a detrimental effect on the physiological status of sick and premature infants, but it appeared to be physiologically beneficial to some of the infants. The mothers who carried out the intervention also appeared to gain from the experience. The results of this study, although small, are felt to be of clinical significance to those working with sick and premature infants and their parents.

RECOMMENDATIONS FOR FUTURE RESEARCH

While attempting to answer the research question cited at the beginning of this study the author became increasingly aware of other areas relating to kangaroo-care which may benefit from further research and investigation. Suggestions for this future research include:

- Clinical trials on lower birth weight and gestation infants ideally beginning at birth.
- An analysis of kangaroo-care on the sleep state of premature and sick infants.
- A comparative study to assess the physiological effect of kangaroo-care and the more traditional cuddle on the infant.
- The effect of kangaroo-care on maternal lactation and breastfeeding would also benefit from further investigation, again especially in premature or low birth weight infants.
- The vast majority of the published work has centred around maternal provision of kangaroo-care; the effect of such care on the father and in turn his infant would also be worthy of study.
- An analysis of maternal/paternal physiological response to kangaroo-care would be of interest.
- Finally, more longitudinally conducted research centred on both the infant and parents may be of benefit in determining long-term outcomes for the child and its family.

REFERENCES

Acolet N, Modi N 1992 Changes in plasma cortisol and catecholamine concentrations in response to massage in pre-term infants. Archives of Disease in Childhood 88: 29–31

Adam K, Oswald I 1984 Sleep helps healing. British Medical Journal 289: 151–162

Affonso D 1989 Reconciliation and healing for mothers through skin to skin contact provided in an American tertiary level Intensive Care Unit. Neonatal Network 12(3): 25–32

Affonso D 1992 Stressors reported by mothers of hospitalized premature infants. Neonatal Network 11(6): 63–70

Anders T F, Keener M 1985 Developmental course of night time sleep–wake patterns in full term and premature infants. Sleep 1(8): 141–147

Anderson G C 1989 Skin to skin: kangaroo care in western Europe. American Journal of Nursing 89(5): 662–666

Armstrong D 1987 Mothers' reaction to kangaroo-care. Infant Behaviour and Development 4: 23–25

Beaver P K 1987 Premature infants' responses to touch and pain: can nurses make a difference? Neonatal Network 6(3): 13–17

Bell F F, Gray J C, Weinstein W R 1980 The effect of thermal balance on the heat balance and insensible water loss in low birthweight infants. Journal of Pediatrics 96: 452–459

Blackburn S 1982 The Neonatal Intensive Care Unit: a high risk environment. American Journal of Nursing 82(11): 1708–1712

Bosque E M 1988 Continuous physiological measures of kangaroo-care versus incubator care in a tertiary level nursery. Pediatric Research 4(2): 402

Brooke O G 1973 Energy retention, energy expenditure and growth in healthy immature infants. Pediatric Research 13: 215–220

Budin P 1907 The nursling. Caxton, London

Buetow K, Klein S 1964 Effect of maintenance of 'normal' skin temperature on survival of infants of low birth weight. Pediatrics 34: 163

Cunningham N, Anisfield E 1987 Infant carrying, breast feeding and mother infant relations (letter). Lancet 1: 379

Cusson R M, Lee A L 1994 Parental intervention on the development of the preterm infant. Journal of Obstetric, Gynecological and Neonatal Nursing 23(1): 60–68

Darnall R A 1987 The thermophysiology of the newborn. Medical Instrument 21: 16–22

De Leeuw R, Edgar C M, Dunnebier E A, Mirmiran M 1991 Physiological effects of kangaroo care in very small preterm infants. Biology of the Neonate 59: 149–155

Detterman D K 1978 The effect of heart beat sound on neonatal crying. Infant Behaviour and Development 1: 36–48

Drosten-Brooks F 1993 Kangaroo care: skin to skin contact in the NICU. M. C. N. 18: 250–253

Glass L 1968 Effects of thermal environment on cold resistance and growth of small infants after the first week of life. Pediatrics 41: 1033–1046

Gorski P A, Davidson M F, Brazelton T B 1983 Direct computer recordings of premature infants and nursery care. Pediatrics 72: 198–202

Graziani L J 1986 Neonatal neurosonograph correlates of cerebral palsy in preterm infants. Pediatrics 78: 17–19

Grimwade J C, Walker D W, Wood C 1970 Sensory stimulation of the human fetus. Australian Journal of Mental Retardation 2: 63–64

Hamlin K, Ramachandran C 1993 Kangaroo care. Canadian Nurse 7: 15–17

Harmon R J 1981 The perinatal period: infants and parents. In: Spittell J A, Brody E (eds) Clinical medicine. Harper and Row, New York

Harrison L L, Leeper J D, Yoon M 1990 Effect of early parental touch on infant heart rates and arterial oxygen saturation levels. Journal of Advanced Nursing 15: 877–885

Horsley A 1988 The neonatal environment. Pediatric Nursing 2: 17–19

Kaplan D M, Mason E A 1960 Maternal reaction to premature birth viewed as an acute emotional disorder. American Journal of Orthopsychiatry 30: 539–552

Klaus M H, Kennell J H 1976 Human maternal and paternal behavior. C V Mosby, St Louis

Klaus M H, Kennell J H 1982 Parent infant bonding. C V Mosby, St Louis

Kling P 1988 Nursing interventions to decrease the risk of periintraventricular/intraventricular haemorrhage. Neonatal Network 11(6): 457–464

Korner A F, Schneider P, Forrest T 1983 Effects of vestibular proprioceptive stimulation on the neurobehavioral development of preterm infants. Neuropediatrics 14: 170–175

Korones S B 1976 Disturbances of infants rest. In: Moore T D (ed) Iatrogenic problems of neonatal intensive care. Ross Labs, Columbus

Lawhorn 1988 Developmental supportive nursing interventions. Paper presented at the 4th Annual Meeting of the National Association of Neonatal Nurses, Chicago

Lawton G, Melzer A 1988 Developmental care of the very low birth weight infant. Journal of Perinatal and Neonatal Nursing 2(1): 56–61

Long J G 1980 Excessive handling as a cause of hypoxia. Pediatrics 65(2): 203–207

Luddington-Hoe S M 1990 Energy conservation during skin-to-skin contact between premature infants and their mothers. Heart and Lung 19(5): 445–451

Maslow A 1970 Motivation and personality. Harper and Row, New York

Merenstein G, Gardner S 1993 Handbook of neonatal intensive care. Mosby, St Louis

Mok Q et al 1991 Temperature instability during nursing procedures in preterm neonates. Archives of Diseases in Childhood 66: 783–786

Norris S, Campbell L, Brenkert S 1981 Nursing procedures and alterations in transcutaneous O2 tension in premature infants. Nursing Research 3: 330–336

Pederson D R 1987 Maternal emotional responses to preterm birth. American Journal of Orthopsychiatry 57(1): 15–21

Perehudoff B 1990 Parents' perceptions of environmental stressors in the special care nursery. Neonatal Network 9(2): 39–44

Picton-Warlow C G, Meyer F E 1970 Cardiovascular response to postural changes in the neonate. Archives of Disease in Childhood 45: 354–359

Polit D F, Hungler B P 1987 Nursing research – principles and methods, 3rd edn. Lippincott, Philadelphia

Rey E S, Martinez H G 1979 Rational management of the premature infant. Paper presented at the First Course of Fetal and Neonatal Medicine. Bogotá, Colombia, March 17–19

Roberton N 1991 A manual of neonatal intensive care. Edward Arnold, London

Roberton N 1992 Textbook of neonatology. Churchill Livingstone, London

Rode S 1981 Attachment patterns of infants separated at birth. Developmental Psychology 17(2): 188–191

Ross G S 1980 Low birth weight babies. Family repercussions. Clinics in Perinatology 7: 47

Sauer P J J 1984 New standards for neutral thermal environment of healthy very low birth weight infants in one week of life. Archives of Disease in Childhood 59: 18–22

Seashore M J 1981 Newborns and parents. Lawrence Erlbaum, Hillsdale

Silverman W A 1987 The 'hands-on or hands-off?' dilemma revisited. Journal of Perinatology 8(4): 277–278

Sloan N L, Camacho L, Rojas E P, Stern C 1994 Kangaroo mother method: randomised controlled trial of an alternative method of care for stabilised low-birthweight infants. Lancet 344: 782–785

Sluckin W 1983 Maternal bonding. Blackwell, Oxford

Speidel B D 1978 Adverse effects of routine procedures on infants. Lancet i: 864–866

Sugarman M 1977 Perinatal influences on maternal–infant attachment. American Journal of Orthopsychiatry 47: 407

Svejda M J 1980 Mother–infant bonding. Child Development 51: 775–779

Trause M A, Kramer L I 1983 The effects of premature birth on parents and their relationship. Developmental Medicine and Child Neurology 25: 459–465

Tucker-Catlett A, Holditch-Davis D 1990 Environmental stimulation of the acutely ill premature infant: physiological effects and nursing implications. Neonatal Network 8(6): 19–26

Volpe J J 1993 Neurosurgery of the newborn. W B Saunders, Philadelphia

Wahlberg V 1992 A retrospective study using the kangaroo method as a complement to standard incubator care. European Journal of Public Health 2(1): 34–37

Watt J E, Strongman K T 1985 The organisation and stability of sleep states in full term, preterm and small for gestational age infants. Developmental Psychology 18: 173–192

Weibley T 1989 Inside the incubator. American Journal of Nursing 14(2): 96–100

Weiss S 1979 The language of touch. Nursing Research 28(2): 76–80

Whitelaw A, Sleath K 1985 Myth of the marsupial mother: home care of very low birth weight infants in Bogotá, Colombia. Lancet 1(1): 1206–1208

Whitelaw A, Heisterkamp G, Sleath K, Acolet D, Richards M 1988 Skin-to-skin contact for very low birth weight infants and their mothers. Archives of Disease in Childhood 63: 1377–1381

Woodson R H, Field T, Greenberg R 1983 Estimating neonatal oxygenation consumption from heart rate. Psychophysiology 20: 558–561

Zeanach C H, Conger C, Jones J D 1984 Clinical application of to traumatized parents: psychotherapy in the intensive care nursery. Child Psychiatry and Human Development 14: 158

The readability of patient information

Duncan Goodes

Commentary

Go into almost any GP surgery, outpatient clinic or hospital ward and you are likely to be greeted by a bank of leaflets and brochures on a diverse range of health education and health restoration topics such as healthy eating and drinking, cardiac rehabilitation, breastfeeding, testicular self-examination and immunization regimes.

Such information giving is, and always will be, a central part of the nurse's role in every setting and nurses often supplement verbal information with written. Whether commercially produced, such as the British Heart Foundation literature, or specially constructed by the nurses in a particular area, the design of such information is critically important.

At a recent seminar, an occupational therapist presented the results of a study of personalized patient information packs. The study looked at the relationships between information, information presentation and information understanding and utilization. The researcher concluded that improving content and presentation increases satisfaction but reduces, at a certain point, understanding and use.

One way of assessing content and presentation is readability, and that is what this chapter covers. Duncan Goodes has identified that it is important to estimate the 'readability' of patient information literature, explored how patient-friendly some of this literature might be, and in particular tested one widely available booklet. He found that it was relatively easy to estimate the readability of the booklet by exposing it to a computer generated test that, with the growth in popularity of home and business computers, is easily accessible by most.

In this chapter Duncan has shown how a topic, that of patient information giving, can be viewed from a new and innovatory perspective, how relatively small-scale research can effectively explore an area and, most importantly perhaps, that we should all pay attention to the readability of the literature that we, as nurses, create. (Readers might be interested to know that this Commentary has readability scores of 28.4 (Flesch), 14 (Flesch-Kincaid Grade level) and 11.5 (Bormuth grade) – read on to find out more!)

Hospital inpatients are being given increasing amounts of written material in support of verbal information. A suitable level of readability has been identified as a key component of successful written material. However, many authors have noted that most patient education literature is at a reading level above the average ability of the population. This study sought to establish the readability of a popular postmyocardial infarction text and to subsequently alter the text to improve its readability. Both the original and the altered text were presented to patients. The effect of this alteration on the postmyocardial infarction patient's perception of the text was assessed by means of a questionnaire.

Questionnaires were returned from 38 patients; however, 11 questionnaires were lost to the study. Of the 27 responses analysed, 15 were from patients who received an altered text and 12 the original. Questionnaires were analysed utilizing statistical methods. The hypothesis generated was that raising the readability index as measured on the Flesch Reading Ease Scale would result in an increase in favourable responses when patients commented on the literature. Statistical analysis of the questionnaires did not support the hypothesis as no significant difference was found between the group receiving the original and that receiving the altered text. It was noted subjectively that nurses reported more favourable comments from those patients receiving the altered text despite findings from questionnaires. The study raises some interesting questions and is of value in identifying future areas of potential research.

INTRODUCTION

The use of patient information literature has become an increasingly universal practice over the last few years. Theoretically there are many advantages to the use of the written word. Oral communication may fail for a number of reasons: it may be misunderstood, forgotten or be given in a situation that is less than ideal for both the giver and the receiver. This latter point is particularly relevant to the nurse/patient situation where the nurse may have to fit an information-giving session into an already busy schedule and have limited choice as to the environment in which it is conducted.

Written information may be produced in such a way as to provide a clear, concise, unambiguous and 'revisitable' resource for the patient. It has been suggested that health carers are more likely to comply with the giving of written information than they are to reliably give verbal information (Ley 1988). The purpose of informing the patient may be to facilitate self-care or foster informed choice as well as increasing the patient's sense of being a valued member of the caring team. This is exemplified by Stephens (1992) who stated that:

Given the trend of 'quicker and sicker' hospital discharges, the patient is required to recuperate at home and assume self-care much more quickly than in the past. The printed materials available for patients must be matched to the reading and comprehension levels of the individual patients.

The demand for improved information has risen with patient expectations of care being given in a partnership between carer and 'caree' and of consent being informed. Patients now expect to be actively involved in the decision-making process. The nurse as an educator will often seek to supplement verbal teaching with written information that summarizes, reinforces or extends the scope of the material given verbally. Printed material remains the most cost-effective and accessible means of giving a permanent resource to the patient. Although magnetic media such as audio and video cassettes are being used in some areas and will, no doubt, become increasingly widespread, it is unlikely that they will totally replace paper media in patient education. The use of printed material has limitations, these mainly being that if learning objectives have been set they may not be achieved if the material is inappropriate for one reason or another. It also has to be recognized that written material is not always the method of choice or, in some cases, an appropriate tool in the achievement of some learning goals. An example would be the teaching of a motor skill or learning visual identification. It is, however, rated well as a means of imparting factual information and in developing desirable attitudes or opinions (Luther & Allensworth 1986).

Assuming that the material given to the patient is appropriate to their condition, the major factor in determining its effectiveness is the accessibility of the text to the reader. This may be described as the readability of the text, with readability being subdivided into three distinct concepts: legibility; ease of reading due to interest value or the pleasantness of the writing; and the ease of comprehension of the material (Luther & Allensworth 1986). There are a number of internationally recognized readability scales. Many of these rely on an understanding of the American schooling system. However, one which does not is the 'Flesch Reading Ease Score' in which a score between 1 and 100 is attributed to a piece of text: the higher the score, the easier it is to read.

Many authors have stressed the importance of readability when considering the suitability of written materials. Likewise, many studies have assessed the readability of various information texts on offer to patients. The conclusion of many of these studies is that the materials on offer are, by and large, too difficult to read to be of use to a substantial portion of the population at which the material is aimed (Lindeman 1988). After a review of a sample of these studies it was felt that an assumption was being made in some cases. It is implied that if the readability index of a piece of information is low (i.e. the piece is difficult to read) then raising it would increase the effectiveness of that information, extend its accessibility to a greater proportion of the target population and increase that population's satisfaction with the material. Whilst this assumption is axiomatic when considering the theory of readability, it appears untested in a 'real world' situation. This study sought to ascertain whether raising the readability index of a piece of published patient information in use nationally would provide a demonstrable benefit to patients.

LITERATURE REVIEW

Studies into the efficacy of written information fall into three broad groups:

1. those that have compared written information with no alternative;
2. those that have compared written information with verbal information;
3. those that have compared verbal information with the use of combined verbal and written information.

Raleigh & Odtohan (1987) reviewed the effects of patient teaching with written material compared with a similar amount of time spent in nurse/patient interaction but with no formal teaching element. They revealed that those patients who received teaching with written information were able to demonstrate, in the short term, increased knowledge and in the long term a sustained and appropriate change in behaviour following myocardial infarction. Duryee (1992) reviewed 14 research papers relating to the efficacy of patient education following myocardial infarction. He reached the conclusion that the papers collectively demonstrated that, in terms of outcome, the best form in which information may be given is verbal, supported or supplemented by text. Those studies that have compared verbal information alone with written information alone reveal little difference between the two in efficacy (Rahe et al 1975). It would appear that the whole is greater than the sum of the parts if an integrated verbal plus written information package is given to the patient. Gauld (1981) compared a control group receiving teaching but no literature with a second group that received literature in support of verbal information. The second group had better knowledge, compliance and behaviour change. However, this outcome has not been universally demonstrated (Morris & Halperin 1979).

Nonetheless the point made earlier that written information is effective in supporting verbal information holds true. This seems to be most particularly true when one considers those patients who have undergone an event that will result in a long-term effect upon their lives. The study by Pozen (1977) perhaps best demonstrates the efficacy of the verbal plus written literature approach to patient education. The study sample consisted of 102 patients admitted to a coronary care unit who were randomly assigned to two groups. One group received the 'usual care' from the coronary care staff; the other received one-to-one sessions supported by written information. A long-term follow-up was conducted and those patients in the second group showed marked improvement in terms of compliance, risk-avoiding behaviours and in return to employment. The difference was found to be most marked in relation to those patients in each group who had been designated 'high risk'. This finding is congruent with the findings of Young & Humphrey (1985) who studied a number of hysterectomy patients and found that those who had received a booklet required less analgesia and were discharged earlier than the control group who did not receive the booklet. It has been stated that: 'No teaching materials negate the need for personal instruction; review the material with the patient, point out the areas that do not apply and reinforce those that do' (Rankin 1984). This statement is well supported by the evidence.

Do patients read written information?

Ley (1988) reviewed the available studies relating to the frequency with which patients stated they had read their health promotion literature. It was demonstrated that between 41% and 95% (mean 72%) of patients will state they have read the literature they have been given. In a similar study Lindeman (1988) undertook a review of research and found that health education material exceeded the reading ability of between 30% and 78% of the sampled populations. Thus, although patients may read health promotion literature, evidence is available that suggests a considerable proportion of the population exposed to written material finds it difficult or impossible to understand.

What is readability?

The term 'readability' predates Flesch (1948), although his work represents the first 'scientific' investigation of the issue of whether text had been written in such a way as to be easy to read. His writings from the 1940s are still regarded as standard works in this area and indeed little has been added to the field that substantially alters the views that he put forward. There are three main constituents to readability, any of which, if deficient, will reduce the value of the text in terms of the benefit it might offer its target population. They are:

1. *Legibility* – when considering printed or typewritten material, this includes consideration of typeface (font), size of type (measured as point value or characters per inch), line spacing, length of printed line (short lines being easier to read; hence newspapers use columns), paragraph spacing, the contrast between print and paper and the quality (sharpness) of the print.

2. *Ease of reading* – either due to interest/relevance to the individual (even a poor reader may spend a long time working with difficult text if they feel it is of value to them) or style (Luther & Allensworth 1986). This is affected by sentence length, punctuation, balance between long words and short words and the use of so-called 'action words' – generally verbs.

3. *Ease of comprehension of the contents* – balance between common and uncommon words and number of syllables per sentence.

Readability formulas are designed to assess the readability of text and may be calculated 'manually' or by computer software. It is important to note that whilst the formulae may very adequately assess the last two components of readability as outlined above, they cannot assess legibility. Whether a text is legible or not is a subjective judgement. It is possible for text to be legible to one person and not to another: for example, with the poorly sighted. Legibility has been subject to guidelines from many sources. Also formulae cannot test an aspect of text that is treated as a separate issue to readability but is allied to it, that is 'comprehensibility' or the ease with which the text may be understood. When considering health information literature substantial portions of the populations being targeted are likely to be in one of two groups: either young or ageing. Both of these groups have special needs. For the purpose of this work only adults are being considered.

Guidelines for legibility

Silver (1991) and Walsh (1991) make a number of suggestions concerning the production of written patient information. These are paraphrased as:

- Text should be in a serif font of at least 14 points if the target population is likely to be over the age of 40 years.
- 1½ spacing is desirable and an A5 format is considered ideal.
- Black print on off-white paper is recommended, provided the paper is not 'glossy' as this causes glare and reflections that hamper reading.
- Type should be lower case except when upper case is the norm, as at the beginning of sentences, for example.
- Ideal line length is said to be 1½ times the length of the alphabet when typed in the chosen font.
- Gaps in the text and graphics break up a potentially daunting mass of words.

Ease of reading

It has been suggested above that the greater the interest a piece of work has for an individual the more likely they are to persevere with reading it even if the text is difficult. Whilst this may be so, there is also evidence that the stress of an acute illness will reduce the reading ability and comprehension of the individual significantly (Kasprisin et al 1992). Readability estimates do not necessarily provide a good indicator of the ease with which text may be comprehended. An example of this might be the work of the poet Edward Lear who produced work that, whilst of a high readability index, is nonetheless difficult to comprehend and has been termed nonsense. This is, however, contrived and Owen et al (1993b) found that when reviewing health education literature, 'readability scores were inversely correlated; that is, the higher the readability score, the lower the comprehension'. It should be noted that the readability formulae they were quoting related to the American school grading system: therefore the higher the scores were, the lower the readability indices would be if one were to apply a Flesch score. Thus for the purposes of this work (using the Flesch Reading Ease Score) this might be paraphrased 'the lower the reading ease, the lower will be the comprehension level'.

This contention may be supported by the finding of a consistently high reliability between the most frequently used formulae (Luther & Allensworth 1986, Meade & Smith 1991, Owen et al

1993a). Merritt et al (1993) found differences between the scores that three different readability formulae produced for a given piece of text although the relative under- or overscoring was consistent between them. The reason for this finding is that some readability scores allocate a schooling grade at which 50% of persons educated to that level would be able to read and access the text. Others allocate a grade at which there would be an expectation of 100% ability. Thus the score (grade allocated) for the first would be lower than the second. Using the Flesch Reading Ease Score overcomes such difficulties as the score given relates to a defined scale of difficulty and percentiles of population expected to be able to read the text. Furthermore, it has been found that many Americans have a reading ability one, two or even three grades below the schooling level claimed to have been achieved (Hussey & Gilliland 1989, Streiff 1986). Although there was no evidence that this is the case in the UK, there was also none to refute it. Therefore using schooling as a measure of reading ability in order to target information to patients may well result in them receiving information that has a reading level above their ability.

Computers and readability estimation

As has been indicated above, readability estimation is, essentially, performed by the application of mathematical formulae. This being the case, there exists an obvious potential for the development of computer software designed to take the drudgery out of performing an estimation. Programs designed for this purpose for use on personal computers (PCs) have developed alongside wordprocessing applications since the early days of PCs in the 1980s. Many such programs will produce a variety of reports utilizing several readability formulae and also offer 'advice' on writing style or on how to improve the readability of the text being analysed. As Meade & Wittbrot (1988) pointed out, performing a similar level of analysis manually would take hours compared with the minutes or even seconds it would take using a PC. However, before a computer can be used to analyse text a sample of that text has to be typed to disk; clearly this is unnecessary with manual methods. If analysis of a very long piece (or many short pieces) was required, the use of a hand scanner and optical character recognition software would become a viable alternative to manual typing of the text. Typically the software will demand a minimum of 100 words or 10 sentences before analysis is possible. The greater the proportion of the text offered to the program for analysis, the greater will be the accuracy of the report if generalizing to the whole of the text is desired. However, when sampling text, standard practice is to take 10 sentences from the beginning of the text, 10 from the middle and 10 from the end (Spadero 1983).

Utilizing a software package is likely to have several advantages: it is time saving, increased accuracy due to absence of human error is likely, high reliability and high validity can be argued, constant reviewing of progress when modifying text by rerunning analysis is enabled and the systematic method facilitates the standardizing of reports for comparative purposes (Kasprisin et al 1992, Meade & Byrd 1989, Meade et al 1992, Meade & Wittbrot 1988).

Patient information

Written educational materials derive from many sources and take many forms. They may be booklets, pamphlets, charts or drug instruction inserts, from single sheets to near books. They may be developed by commercial companies, charitable organizations, hospitals or individuals. The information may be a photocopy of handwritten notes or a professionally produced product. The one common element within this seemingly disparate collection is that they all seek to serve a common purpose and that is to increase the knowledge of the target population (and possibly change behaviour) either in their own right or as an adjunct to verbal or other visual information.

Since the work of Hayward (1975) there has been a growing assumption that patients will benefit from information; any information. Many studies have shown that patients are strongly in favour of receiving a permanent record of information regarding their condition or treatment (Gauld 1981, Mazis et al 1978). In addition, it has been shown that the level of satisfaction with information is directly proportional to the amount of information given (Mazis et al 1978, Morris & Kanouse 1980). However, if a patient is to benefit from written information a number of prerequisites have to be met. These are that: 'To be effective written information has to be noticed, read, understood, believed and remembered' (Ley 1988). If the material the patients are expected to learn from is inaccessible, difficult to read or to understand or the patients are disinclined to believe it, it is unlikely to be of benefit to them.

Meade & Wittbrot (1988) go further than this and state that:

Materials that are above a patient's reading level may become a health hazard for the patient and also a liability for the health professional if important information has been distributed but not understood.

Similarly, Meade & Smith (1991) have stated that: Reading material that is written above the reading level of patients is useless and contributes to loss of time and money.

Readability of patient information

If patients are to fully understand the written material with which they are presented then it must be written at a readability level within their reading ability. This is the foundation on which the concepts of readability are based. Many studies have been conducted to assess the readability of patient information. In order to interpret these studies (all of which were conducted in North America) in context with this study, refer to Table 3.1 which equates a Flesch Reading Ease Score with an American schooling grade. Collectively, the eight studies that were reviewed sampled 184 patient information texts. The readability formula used for the studies was either the Gunning Fog Index (Gunning 1952), the SMOG formula (McLaughlin 1969) or both. The high number of studies utilizing the SMOG formula suggests that this will become the standard measure of the readability of patient information in America. SMOG produces a grade level at which 100% of those persons schooled to that level would be expected to understand the text; therefore its scores tend to be 1–2 grades higher than that of the Fog Index which assumes that 50% of those educated to the specified grade would understand the piece of text. Table 3.2 summarizes the studies reviewed.

The average reading ability of North Americans is said to be around 8th grade (Boyd & Citro 1983). From the studies reviewed it can be seen that much of the literature sampled exceeded the

Table 3.1 Comparing Flesch Reading Ease Scores with American school grades (after Spadero, 1983)

Flesch Reading Ease Score	School grade	Syllables per 100 words	Average sentence length (words)
90–100	5	123	8
80–90	6	131	11
70–80	7	139	14
60–70	8–9	147	17
50–60	10–12	155	21
30–50	College	167	25
0–30	University	192	29

Table 3.2 Summary of findings from studies investigating the readability of patient information

Reference	Number of texts reviewed	Specialism	Average grade
Merrit et al 1993	4	Hypercholest-erolaemia	SMOG 13
Evanoski 1990	5	Ventricular tachycardia	Fog 10.4
Meade et al 1992	51	American Cancer Society literature	SMOG 11.9
Larson & Schumacher 1992	15	Arthritis	SMOG 10.9
Bauman et al 1989	9	Asthma	SMOG 11.7
Stephens 1992	8	Cancer	SMOG 10.4
Owen et al 1993a	37	Cardiac	Fog 12.2
Spadero 1983	55	Child/family	SMOG 10.2

Average grade attributed = 11.3

average ability of the American population to read it. If the text is reconciled with average ability (that is, written at grade 8–9) then by definition, 50% of the population would and 50% of the population would not be fully able to read it. This simple statement makes a target of material being written for average ability questionable as this is to aim for a level at which half the population cannot fully access the material.

Klingelhofer & Gershwin (1988) suggest that: 'an estimated one third of American adults do not comprehend anything beyond the most rudimentary written material'. Nonetheless, it is the gap between the actual reading level of the material tested and the average reading level of the population that many researchers comment upon. It could be contended that this is addressing only half the problem. Evanoski (1990) and Larson & Schumacher (1992) both pick up this point by suggesting that material should be written at a 6th grade level. This is equivalent to a Flesch Reading Ease Score of 80–90. As Visser (1980) pointed out:

How well patients remember written information depends on the level of readability and the limitations of the patient's medical knowledge. The easily readable leaflets lead to more accurate use of medicines, better adherence to dietary rules and greater retention of the information.

Esty et al (1991) reviewed the comprehension levels of patients reading health information. They used two different assessments of patient comprehension and concluded that if a substantial proportion of the population was to understand written information it should be written at no higher than grade 5 level. There is a paucity of information from this side of the Atlantic regarding both population averages and the readability of patient information. Couchman & Dawson (1990) suggested that the average reading ability of the British population is 9 years of age although they do not quote their source for this information. Reviewing three pieces of patient information, two from the British Heart Foundation (BHF) and one from Help for Health (HFH), produced interesting results. The two BHF texts achieved Flesch scores of 47 and 49 and the HFH text 30. Flesch scores of 40–50 indicate that 35–50% of the population can fully access the text and a score of 30 around 15%. Although by no means an exhaustive survey, this suggests that at least some British texts are no more readable than their American counterparts. For illustrative purposes it might be noted that this literature review rates a Flesch Reading Ease Score of 51. It is, therefore, easier to read than some information given to patients for educative purposes.

Cautions and considerations

This body of evidence suggests that the use of readability formulae or, rather, application of the information gained by using the formulae will make written material more valuable. Unfortunately this may not be so. Readability formulae will only assess the syntactic and semantic elements of the texts examined. As has been suggested above, other aspects of text will also affect how useful it is to the target population. Legibility has been mentioned already. Other aspects to consider are accuracy of information, presentation and the prior experience of the reader. Another often overlooked factor is the situation and environment in which the information is going to be read. How many people have struggled with 'flat packed' furniture? Reading the instructions is, for many, something of a last resort; almost an admission of defeat! The reader needs to be receptive, motivated to read the material presented, have time to read the material and possibly needs time to reflect on it if behaviour change is to result. The evidence born of research into the efficacy of differing means of providing patient information strongly supports this latter contention; verbal information is best in the short term and written in the longer term, with a combination being the best approach. Visser (1980) demonstrated that giving a pamphlet presurgery had little beneficial effect over the usual verbal information. Gauld (1981) produced a study underlining the efficacy of supporting verbal information with written. Overall it would appear that one-to-one teaching is the method of choice in 'pre-event' situations (for example, prior to surgery) whereas written information appears to quite specifically benefit those patients who of necessity or desire are proposing a long-term change in lifestyle (for example, post-myocardial infarction).

Alternative media

Although it would seem extremely unlikely that paper will be entirely replaced as a permanent medium for information presentation, there are increasingly viable alternatives. CAL (computer assisted learning) is one such alternative, as are video or audio packages. 'CAL has been demonstrated as being superior to both written and verbal formats in promoting recall and in performance in the undertaking of clinical procedures' (Fisher et al 1977, cited by Noble 1991).

Certainly the interactive, self-paced nature of computer learning is attractive as is the ability to 'go over' material repeatedly without the patient feeling they are wasting someone's valuable time. Clearly with well-written software and the option for the use of voice chips, CAL utilizing magnetic (disk) or optical (CD) media has the potential to overcome many of the difficulties associated with targeting written material to the patient's reading level. The fact that programs can be written in such a way as to obviate the need for computing or keyboard skills can make such packages very user friendly (Luker & Caress 1989). However, it seems that as the patient is unlikely to be able to take such materials home with them, CAL's future may lie in the pre-event (for example, prior to surgery) rather than postevent (for example, poststroke) arena. As such it is, perhaps, more likely to take over from the health carer giving verbal teaching than from paper accompanying the patient home.

THE STUDY

Introduction

The literature review and analysis of some patient information texts highlighted two important points: firstly that an appropriate readability level is considered an important feature of effective patient information and secondly that much patient information has an inappropriate readability level for its target population. In the literature reviewed regarding this topic, there is the implication that should a text with a low readability index be altered to raise that index then patient satisfaction will similarly rise.

This study involved identifying a piece of patient information text with a well-defined target population that was in common usage. The index of the original text was assessed and then the text was altered to raise that index.

A hypothesis was formed that stated:

Raising the Flesch Reading Ease Score of a piece of patient information will increase the incidence of favourable patient responses when they comment on the text.

The hypothesis was tested by allocating patients drawn from the literature's target population to one of two groups, the first receiving the original text and the second an altered text with a higher readability index. Comments were elicited from both groups by the use of a questionnaire and the results analysed to establish whether the alteration had any effect on the patients' perception of the text.

Definition of terms

For the purposes of this study readability is defined as the difficulty attached to the reading of a piece of text as determined by the use of a readability formula (adapted from Owen et al 1993a). The formula is a means of assessing the difficulty of reading a piece of text by analysing the length of sentences, the ratio of common to uncommon words, the average number of syllables in each sentence and the number of polysyllabic words used.

Literature in use nationally

In order to ascertain what information is being used nationally the author firstly sent out 30 letters to hospitals spread nationally. Care was taken to include small and large, rural and urban settings. The letter allowed a member of the hospital's acute medical ward or coronary care unit to identify the written information used for its patients in the recovery period postmyocardial infarction (MI). Stamped self-addressed envelopes accompanied the letters. To facilitate returns the letter had space available on which the staff could record their response and return it. The letters did not identify the hospital to which they had been sent and as such returns were anonymous. After 3 weeks 16 had been returned with a single further response being received after 2 months. All the units responding used British Heart Foundation (BHF) literature. Of the BHF literature used, all units listed booklet No. 1 *Back to Normal* amongst others. Of the 17 responding units only three identified 'in house' material as contributing to the information given to patients. As it was clear that *Back to Normal* is in widespread use this text was chosen for the study. A letter was sent to the head office of the BHF informing them of the study and seeking permission to critically analyse their text and subsequently alter it with a view to presenting it to patients for comment. A reply was received expressing an interest in the work, giving permission for the use of BHF literature and indicating a desire to see the results.

Assessing the readability of text

The text of *Back to Normal* was typed to computer disk, formatted as a text file and analysed for readability by the use of three software programs. The programs used were:

1. Grammatik 5
2. Readability Plus
3. Correct Grammar.

Three programs were used in order to assess whether they produced consistent reports. It was found that the scores produced by the three programs varied by less than 5% and that the Readability Plus program most closely reconciled with a manual assessment of a 20-sentence, 249-word piece of text. The scale chosen for the study as a measure of readability was the Flesch Reading Ease Score as this score is interpreted by relating to standard text types rather than the American schooling grade system. The Flesch Reading Ease formula is determined as follows:

Reading ease = 206.835 − 0.846W − 1.015S where W is the average number of syllables per 100 words and S is the average sentence length in words.

The formula produces a score 20 and 90 for 'real' text (out of a possible range 0–100). It would be possible to construct text that fell outside the expected range of results but it would have to be obviously contrived. Table 3.3 gives further meaning to the Flesch Reading Ease Scores.

The original text of the *Back to Normal* booklet rated a Flesch Reading Ease Score of 49. Following alteration to the text the score was raised to 63. This should increase the percentage of people able to fully understand the text from around 35–50% to 77–82%. Another way to view this increase is to consider that about 60% of people who could not fully access the original material would now be able to do so. An example of an original paragraph and its altered form are given below for comparative purposes.

Table 3.3 Meaning of Flesch Reading Ease Scores

Score	Description	Typical example	% of population able to fully access
90–100	Very easy	Child's book	95–97
80–90	Easy	Pulp fiction	88–95
70–80	Fairly easy	Popular fiction	82–90
60–70	Average	Magazines	77–82
50–60	Fairly hard	Classic novels	50–77
40–50	Difficult	Specialist articles	35–50
30–40	Hard	Academic texts	15–35
20–30	Very hard	Scientific papers	< 15

Original text from *Back to Normal*

In a heart attack (or coronary thrombosis) one of the coronary arteries that supply blood to the heart muscle becomes blocked off by a clot; the part of the heart muscle that this artery supplies becomes starved of oxygen and is damaged. This usually causes severe pain in the chest which may last for hours, but other symptoms may include nausea, vomiting, faintness and breathlessness. It may also produce disturbances in the rhythm of the heart and, if the damage to the muscle is extensive, the heart may fail in its job of providing enough blood for the body to function properly. Although the heart attack is often a sudden and dramatic event, it is the result of a process that has been going on for many years. Narrowing of the coronary arteries starts in youth or early adult life, and is due to a gradual deposition of fatty substances in the lining of the blood vessel. The wall of such a diseased artery may crack; blood cells called 'platelets' become attached to the area. A clot (or 'thrombus') composed of fibrous material called 'fibrin' may form on top of this, which may partly or completely block the artery. If the heart muscle cells supplied by this artery are deprived of oxygen for more than a few minutes they may die, causing what is called a 'myocardial infarction', 'myocardial' referring to the heart muscle and 'infarction' to its death. Usually the amount of muscle damaged is small and once the attack is over, there is enough good muscle left for the heart to do its work satisfactorily.

Altered text from *Return to Normal*

In a heart attack one of the blood vessels that supply blood to the heart muscle becomes blocked off by a clot. The part of the heart muscle that this artery supplies becomes starved of oxygen and is damaged. This usually causes severe pain in the chest which may last for hours. Other symptoms may include feeling sick, being sick, faintness and breathlessness. It may also disturb the beating of the heart. If a lot of muscle is damaged, the heart may not be able to provide enough blood for the body. Although the heart attack often happens suddenly, it is the result of a process that has been going on for many years. Narrowing of the coronary arteries starts in youth or early adult life. It is due to a slow build-up of fat in the lining of the blood vessel. The wall of the artery may crack. Blood cells called 'platelets' become attached to the damaged area. A clot may form on top of this, which may partly or completely block the artery. If the heart muscle supplied by this artery is short of oxygen for more than a few minutes it may die. This results in what is called a heart attack or 'myocardial infarction'. 'Myocardial' refers to the heart muscle and 'infarction' to its death. Usually the amount of muscle damaged is small and once the attack is over, there is plenty of good muscle left for the heart to do its job.

This increase in reading ease reflects simple changes to the text; decreasing the number of polysyllabic words, substituting common words for uncommon ones and shortening sentence length. It has been suggested that the removal of polysyllabic medical terminology is a means of improving the readability of patient information (Owen et al 1993a). It was decided not to take this route as, although a further improvement in readability would have undoubtedly resulted, the same authors point out that most patients cannot accurately define even monosyllabic medical terms. Thus it was decided to retain medical terms with an explanation of their meaning. Patients are going to hear or read such terms and it was felt that a 'dictionary' function within the written information would be important. Using this approach it is believed that a further significant improvement in the readability of the *Back to Normal* text would be difficult to achieve as the limiting factor becomes those medical terms being present.

The text was reproduced in two forms both utilizing the original graphics and format (that is, line length, paragraph spacing, paragraph headings and use of bold and italicized fonts). One copy retained the original text, font and title, the other featured modified text to raise the readability index and a larger serif font to enhance legibility. This second copy was retitled *Return to Normal*. Every effort was made to ensure that the only differences between the two were those measures taken to improve readability reflected in *Return to Normal*.

Aims of the research

The research was undertaken to establish if, as has been implied by many authors, raising the readability index of a piece of patient information text would increase the quality of that text from the patients' perspective. The quality of the text would be defined by indicators which were to be reported upon by the 'end-user', namely the patient. The researcher sought to ascertain if theoretical benefits pertained to the 'real world'. A hypothesis was formed:

Raising the Flesch Reading Ease Score of a piece of patient information will increase the incidence of favourable patient responses when they comment on the text.

Thus the independent variable manipulated was the readability of the text and the dependent variable the response to that change. By the application of a quantitative approach and the definition of these two variables, statistical analysis of the relationship between them would be possible.

Questionnaire design

The work of Luther & Allensworth (1986) in the development of a Reading Material Checklist was valuable in identifying the key features of written materials. It has been argued that for written information to be effective it has to be 'noticed, read, understood, believed and remembered' (Ley 1988). Additionally health information should be deemed to have utility for the reader and should result in a change in behaviour (Merritt et al 1993). Both Rankin (1984) and Meade & Byrd (1989) define a role for reinforcing verbal information. Thus it might be hoped that reading a piece of health information literature might enable the reader to better participate in interaction with their health carers. Owen et al (1993b) state that 'personalization' of text is important, meaning that the text should be written in such a way that the reader feels it is talking about them and their situation rather than some abstract of life in general. The use of a 14-point serif font to aid legibility is suggested by Silver (1991) and Walsh (1991). By utilizing the indicators described a set of questions was drawn together as a blueprint for a questionnaire that would test whether the indicators had been achieved with a high degree of validity. In the introductory section in the questionnaire respondents were asked to identify their age, gender and the name of the booklet they read.

The questions

Seven questions were devised that would test whether the indicators applied to the piece of text. Four further questions sought the reader's subjective opinion of the text and one question was included to check the consistency of the respondents' scoring. Questions were so constructed as to vary the 'favourable' response between yes and no. The 'check' question was as follows:

No 4. Was the booklet called *Back to Normal*? (Any return in which the answer to this question did not reconcile with the title the patient had given for the name of the booklet they had read was to be declared lost data.)

The following lists show the number order in which the questions appeared.

Indicator questions:

1. Did you read all of the booklet?
2. Will you refer to it again?
3. Will it be useful when you go home?
5. Did you have to reread parts of the booklet to understand it?
6. Did you find parts of the content irrelevant?
9. Did the booklet make you feel you could ask the doctors and nurses more informed questions after you had read it?

Opinion questions:

7. Would you change the contents if you had the chance?
8. Was the booklet too complicated?
11. Do you think there was too much jargon in the booklet?
12. Do you think it could be made easier to read?

Additionally nine statements were constructed with the respondents being asked to rank their response on a 6-point forced choice Likert Scale (see Table 3.4).

The statements themselves were designed to test consistency of scoring and to allow respondents more choice in their response, thus offering a more sensitive measure of the differences perceived between the two pieces of text. A mix of positively and negatively expressed statements was used to avoid inserting a bias in responses (Burns & Grove 1987).

Statement for which response requested:

13. I found the booklet clearly written.
14. There were parts of the booklet I did not understand.
15. I felt it did not talk about my situation.
16. I felt the booklet was sexist in places.

Table 3.4 Likert Scale

1. Totally disagree with the statement.
2. Disagree with the statement.
3. Disagree a little with the statement.
4. Agree a little with the statement.
5. Agree with the statement.
6. Strongly agree with the statement.

17. I found the print easy to read.
18. Reading it will not change what I do when I get home.
19. It was easier to read than my usual reading material.
20. I felt it was too simple.
21. The booklet is useful.

In writing the questionnaire the author ensured that the readability index of the questionnaire was greater than that of the simplest text offered (that is, it was easier to read). There seemed little point in testing the ability of people to understand a text if they could not understand the questions. The questionnaire rated a Flesch Reading Ease Score of 82.

Research setting

The study was conducted (initially) on two acute medical wards in a small general hospital. Both provide inpatient facilities for a broad range of clients in terms of age and presenting condition. Both the wards function as '24-hour on take' units and patients with known or suspected myocardial infarction are admitted direct or via the accident and emergency department. The majority of cardiac admissions are ambulance admissions either as a result of a general practitioner having called an ambulance to the victim's home or as a result of a call from a member of the public. Medical staffing on the wards is provided by three senior house officers and a single house officer: there is no senior medical cover on site. Nursing staffing is at relatively high levels in respect of numbers and skill mix: both wards have senior nurses with coronary care and/or intensive care experience.

Midway through the data collection process it became clear that insufficient data for statistically reliable analysis were going to be generated in the time available for data collection without the use of an additional site. A ward in a large city hospital was identified and permission obtained from senior nursing and medical staff to utilize it for the study. Being within the same authority, the approval of a second ethical committee was not necessary. Medical staffing to registrar level is resident on the hospital site and the nursing staff are all coronary care trained. This area was 'co-opted' to the study.

Patient sample

The sample used for the study was a sample of convenience with any patient admitted with an acute myocardial infarction who was not in an exclusion group being recruited to the study. Patients were not informed of the study prior to the presentation of the questionnaire as this might have influenced the results considerably. The questionnaire offered an introductory explanation in brief and those nurses who undertook to hand questionnaires out were given instructions to pass on to the patient and an explanation of the study. This explanation included the prevention of 'priming the patient' as it was hoped that their responses might be as valid as possible and not be given to 'please the nurse'. The senior member of nursing staff in each of the wards was asked to exercise her judgement on whether there was any patient who might be considered unsuitable on health grounds. In order to 'standardize' the responses only patients who had suffered their first myocardial infarction were included, thus avoiding the influence of previous personal experience.

Exclusions

The following groups of patients were excluded from the study:

1. Any patient who had required resuscitation before or after arrival on the ward.
2. Any patient deemed unfit by a senior nurse.
3. Any non-English-speaking patient.
4. Any patient having had a previous infarction.

Demography of respondents

The demography of the two patient groups is summarized in Table 3.5. It was felt that the two groups were sufficiently similar not to affect the outcome of the study. In particular, the level of schooling of the two groups would not have been affected by the slight age difference between them. Although the *Return to Normal* group is larger than the other, the two groups are, essentially, homogeneous.

Table 3.5 Demography of respondents

	Male	Female	Average age (yrs)
Back to Normal (original text)	10	2	61.2
Return to Normal (altered text)	12	3	63.3

(The *Back to Normal* group included three patients from the large city hospital and the *Return to Normal* group four patients.)

Ethical considerations

At the inception of the study opinions were sought from the consultants with clinical responsibility for patients potentially in the target groups. Consent to conduct the study was gained from the care group general manager and each of the three consultants admitting patients to the clinical areas involved. The senior nursing staff who would be involved were also approached and given an outline of the study itself and potential implications for staff should they agree to assist with data collection at a later date. Due to the author's senior role in the hospital every effort was made to ensure that staff were clear that they were under no duress to agree to requests for assistance with the research. The information sessions proved useful in highlighting some potential problems upon which the author acted. This participation in the process also, perhaps, gave a degree of ownership to staff assisting in data collection. The study was subject to the scrutiny of the ethics committee before data collection commenced. A small pilot study was performed only once approval had been granted. This facilitated the finalizing of the questionnaire design.

Confidentiality and consent

Patient confidentiality was an issue that tied in closely with the researcher's desire for patients' replies to be anonymous. The means of achieving this took considerable thought. The result was a system in which the two different information booklets were placed into numbered envelopes without the envelope being sealed down. The purpose of the numbering was to ensure the two types of booklet were given out in equal numbers and in sequence to overcome as much as possible the influence of changes in staffing patterns or other variables from week to week. Once the patient had had the information for two days he or she was given a questionnaire with instructions that completion was entirely voluntary and that they should seal it into the envelope in which they had originally received their booklet prior to returning it to the nurse. The nurse would assure the patients that the researcher would be the only one to see their reply if they chose to complete the form and that should they choose not to, then the nurse would not know.

The instructions to nursing staff were presented to the clinical areas as a flowchart to which staff might refer should they have any doubts about how to proceed. This promoted consistency in the administration of the questionnaire as an aid to validity (Burns & Grove 1987). Patient confidentiality was ensured by there being no record of patient details in relation to the study kept on the ward areas, questionnaires being identified numerically and being returned anonymously.

The questionnaire itself requested that the patient identify their age and gender only. In addition to the verbal information given to the patient when they were given their questionnaire, the questionnaire included an introduction describing in brief the purpose of the research, the status of the researcher and stressing that participation in terms of completing the questionnaire was voluntary. Reports received from nursing staff on the clinical areas involved suggested that patients were, on the whole, delighted to be asked their opinion.

Pilot studies

The questionnaire was piloted on two occasions, firstly amongst nursing staff and secondly with seven patients. Piloting with nursing staff revealed problems with the rating system for the statements on a visual analogue scale. This was changed to a Likert Scale for the patient pilot.

The second pilot revealed that patients found the completion of a numerical scale after each statement difficult and some 'pattern' scoring was apparent with inconsistent scoring favouring the right-hand end of the scale. For the finalized questionnaire the scale to be used was given in an introductory section with an explanation and example of its use. Scoring required the respondents to put the number that best matched their responses into an empty box after the statement. It was hoped that this would require the patient to check the scale for each response and sought to remove 'patterning'. The use of 'positive' and 'negative' questions made a 'straight 6s or straight 1s' response to questions 13–21 inconsistent and it was decided that should such a response be received it would be declared lost data. The last patient in the pilot group commented favourably on the changes. In addition to changes in the scoring system some questions were refined and two removed as they were likely to produce invalid data. The questions removed attempted to assess comprehension of the material but it was felt unlikely that answers would or could reflect a patient's level of understanding of the text.

Analysis of the data produced

The questionnaire consisted of two types of questions: those answered yes or no and those ranked on the Likert Scale. Additionally some of the questions were asked in positive terms and others in the negative. Negative questions were those questions where 'no' or a ranking of 1 on the Likert Scale were the most favourable responses. In order to standardize the responses on the Likert Scale those questions asked in the negative were identified and the responses were then transposed as if the question had been asked in the positive.

Fisher's Exact Probability Test

The first 12 questions required simple yes/no responses, producing nominal data. The data were arranged into a 2×2 contingency table for each question. The sample size was less than 40, making a straightforward chi-squared analysis inappropriate. As the smallest cell values in the table were less than 5, using a chi-squared analysis with Yates correction was invalid. Thus the Fisher's Exact Probability Test became the method of choice despite the calculation being complex (see Burns & Grove 1987).

t-test for unmatched samples

An unmatched t-test is utilized when the two sets of data are drawn from two different populations (as opposed to two readings from the same population). The test is parametric although for small sample sizes the t distribution rather than the normal distribution is utilized. In respect of questions 13–21 scored on the Likert Scale the values for each item are technically ordinal level data and the summed and averaged scores for each subject interval level data (Burns & Grove 1987 p 319). The summed scores are amenable to the application of the t-test for unmatched samples as the sample is large enough and the two groups reveal homoscedasticity and minimal skew.

RESULTS

Thirty-eight patients participated in the study. Eleven questionnaires were lost to the study for various reasons. Four were lost due to patients being transferred to non-participating sites (2) or being discharged home earlier than expected (2). In three responses the answer to question 4 did not reconcile with the name of the text as identified by the patient: these responses were treated as lost data. One response was returned with a note from ward staff that the patient was blind (!): this was treated as lost data. Two responses revealed wildly inconsistent scoring and were treated as lost data. One patient died prior to completing the questionnaire. Therefore, there were 27 responses available for analysis. Of these, 12 were responses from patients having received *Back to Normal* (the original text) and the remaining 15 from respondents who had received *Return to Normal*.

The results for questions 1–12 are presented in Table 3.6.

Table 3.6   Results for questions 1–12

Question	Booklet	Yes	No	Total	p
1. Did you read all of the booklet?	Back	11	1	12	
	Return	14	1	15	
	Total	25	2	27	0.51*
2. Will you refer to it again?	Back	11	1	12	
	Return	14	1	15	
	Total	25	2	27	0.51*
3. Will it be useful when you go home?	Back	11	1	12	
	Return	14	1	15	
	Total	25	2	27	0.51*
4. Did you have to re-read parts of the booklet to understand it?	Back	5	7	12	
	Return	10	5	15	
	Total	15	12	27	0.136*
5. Did you find parts of the content irrelevant?	Back	1	11	12	
	Return	4	10	14	
	Total	5	21	26	0.182*
6. Would you change the contents if you had the chance?	Back	0	12	12	
	Return	1	14	15	
	Total	1	26	27	0.55*
7. Was the booklet too complicated?	Back	1	11	12	
	Return	0	15	15	
	Total	1	26	27	0.44*
8. Did the booklet make you feel you could ask more informed questions after you had read it?	Back	10	2	12	
	Return	11	4	15	
	Total	21	6	27	0.30*
9. Can you recall what was said about your condition?	Back	12	0	12	
	Return	13	2	15	
	Total	25	2	27	0.30*
10. Do you think there is too much jargon in the booklet?	Back	1	11	12	
	Return	3	12	15	
	Total	4	23	27	0.31*
11. Do you think it could be made easier to read?	Back	1	11	12	
	Return	6	9	15	
	Total	7	20	27	0.07*

Back = *Back to Normal*
Return = *Return to Normal*
* There is no significant difference between groups.

Table 3.7 t-test results

Group	Cases	Mean	Std dev	Std error
Back to Normal	12	4.94	0.505	0.146
Return to Normal	15	4.83	0.4081	0.105
Sample vs. sample		Difference	t-value	df
Back vs. *Return*		0.107	0.774	25

Table 3.8 Second t-test results

Group	Cases	Mean	Std dev	Std error
Back to Normal	9	3.34	1.57	0.52
Return to Normal	9	3.42	1.51	0.50
Sample vs. sample		Difference	t-value	df
Back vs. *Return*		−0.12	0.315	16

Likert scores

For questions 13–21 the mean of the scores for each subject was calculated after transposition of negatively framed questions and the two sets of means were subjected to a t-test for unmatched samples. The results are detailed in Table 3.7. This demonstrates no significant difference between the responses of the two groups of patients.

A further t-test was conducted on the summed and average scores per item (that is, for each question 13–21). Results are detailed in Table 3.8. This demonstrates no significant difference in the responses to each question between groups.

Statistical analysis of the data produced no instances of significant difference in any data set analysed.

Measure of central tendency

Table 3.9 displays a comparison of the mean scores for *Back to Normal* and *Return to Normal* in respect of questions 13–21 answered on the Likert Scale. Scores for negative questions have been transposed.

DISCUSSION

The analysis of the data produced by the questionnaires reveals no significant difference in statistical terms between the two

Table 3.9 Comparison of mean scores for questions 13–21

Question	Back to Normal	Return to Normal
13	5.08	5.00
14	4.16	4.33
15	4.41	4.66
16	5.66	4.78
17	5.08	5.33
18	4.83	4.53
19	4.08	4.13
20	4.91	4.86
21	5.41	5.40

groups. Thus the hypothesis was not supported. That this study found no difference between responses to literature with a Flesch score of 49 and that with a score of 63 was a surprising finding. Several things may account for this. The conclusions drawn from earlier studies could be wrong in their assumption that readability was as significant as they thought. This is extremely unlikely as many studies have been conducted and replicated producing similar data. The tool used may have been insufficiently sensitive as a measure or something was coming into play that was not tested. Lastly, the analysis of the data may have failed to find a difference that exists within the data.

Nursing staff consistently reported that the text with the higher readability was more favourably received. Some patients, having completed the questionnaire, then 'compared notes' with their peers who had received the alternative literature; all favoured the altered text to the extent that some patients who had not originally had it insisted on a copy. Nursing staff themselves also expressed a preference for the altered text. Senior staff also reported that patients who had received the altered text appeared to be better informed and seemed to require less verbal input compared with those receiving the original text.

Therefore, it seems clear that the questionnaire failed in eliciting a response on an aspect of readability that is very important. It could be concluded that this crucially important aspect cannot be one of the areas tested as the preference for the altered text was sufficiently strongly stated and reported to have produced a measurable difference in responses had it been tested for. It should be noted that the materials were presented in such a way as to ensure the only difference between them was the text. Thus some other factor is likely to be involved. The questions are, then:

1. What didn't the questionnaire measure?

2. Is there something within the data that the methods of analysis utilized failed to highlight?

The first question will be discussed at length. In respect of the statistical methodology the use of the Fisher's Exact Probability Test is, in light of the literature and of advice, a robust decision (Bourke et al 1985, Herbet 1990, Rimm & Hartz 1980). However, the use of the t-test for those questions answered on the Likert Scale perhaps presents some problems. The method requires the summing (or summing and averaging) of scores for subjects responding. The values obtained are then analysed. This may hide a difference in response to a single item within the questionnaire, as the test is of 'gross' difference between the respondents' scoring for the two samples. An additional analysis was undertaken to establish by means of a t-test whether there was any difference in the mean score per item as opposed to mean score per respondent. This test also revealed no significant difference. This fact prompted a search for another test that could be applied to the responses at a nominal level without recourse to rendering the data interval level. This, it was hoped, would allow a difference in response to a single item to be identified.

In terms of the measure of central tendency for the scores per item, the modes for each question were identical other than where one item might be bimodal in one group and not in the other and the arithmetic means differed little. Both these findings reflect the homogeneity of the data sets which accounts, in part, for the statistical findings. The conclusion reached is that there truly is no difference between the two sets of responses. The data analysis was rigorous and suitable for the data.

Thus for there to be a preference the questionnaire must have failed as a measuring tool. What doesn't the questionnaire measure? The most obvious feature of the questionnaire is that to be a valid tool it requires the respondent to answer the questions honestly and also critically. Despite the measures taken to combat response bias in the questionnaire design, this may still have affected the data. A patient may perceive a favourable response as desired. This perception may, consciously or unconsciously, colour their responses. Certainly the pilot study revealed inconsistent scoring towards the right-hand end of a scale (see above). As only one score out of both groups and for all questions in the study had a mode of less than 5 (4) it seems possible that patients have scored less critically than they might have. However, this does not explain the comments nurses received and reported.

What doesn't the questionnaire measure? The specific answer

to this is comprehension. It is probable that a questionnaire as a tool to measure comprehension would be extremely difficult to construct if it were not to be both invalid and unreliable. Indeed, questions removed at the pilot stage sought to ascertain the level of the patient's comprehension of the respective texts. They were removed as being invalid (unlikely to consistently test that which they were designed to test). It is interesting to note that in Luther & Allensworth's (1986) 41-point Reading Material Checklist (as resourced at the questionnaire design stage), comprehensibility or patient comprehension of the material gets no mention. It may be worth those utilizing the checklist ensuring that not only is material comprehensive but also comprehensible. It is just possible that all the points identified could apply to a text but comprehensibility be lacking.

To gain valid and reliable data concerning the comprehension levels of readers exposed to text, the best recognized procedure is the Cloze test. In this test the material is presented with the first and last sentences intact but with every fifth word (excluding nouns and pronouns) removed from the remaining sentences with a minimum of 50 blanks. Subjects are requested to fill in the missing words, anything other than an exact replacement being scored as a failure. Ability to understand the text is indicated by scores above 60% success. Scores below 40% indicate inability to comprehend the material. It has been stated earlier that readability has been found to correlate well with comprehension (Owen et al 1993). This has not been universally demonstrated. Holcomb & Ellis (1978) conducted Cloze tests on American Heart Association information and found that comprehension levels were 'significantly lower' than the readability level of the text. It is possible that patients found the altered text as used in this study more acceptable not because it was more readable (the aspect of the text about which they had been asked to respond) but because it was more comprehensible – something they were not given the opportunity to comment upon.

In general terms the way in which the study was conducted proved successful. The measures taken to ensure standardization of procedure and to maintain patient confidentiality were effective and 'minimally invasive' in terms of disrupting staff or patient routines. The main conclusion to be drawn from this study is that readability as such is but one aspect of successful literature. It is possible that the reasons patients (or anyone else for that matter) find literature accessible and useful are more complex than at first thought and are to a degree subjective. This being the case, a qualitative rather than quantitative approach may have elicited more useful data. Clearly 'something is going on' that made the altered text more acceptable. Research questions that start from an 'I know something is going on but not what' standpoint lend themselves to a grounded theory (Glaser & Strauss 1967) approach and patient interviews. Comprehensibility is a factor that was not sufficiently considered at the inception of the project but is, as a result of the findings, now thought to be potentially of substantial importance. Patients scored both texts highly, perhaps reflecting the desirability of offering literature to patients in support of verbal instructions. All patients bar one felt the literature they received to be valuable and likely to be of use to them when they returned home. This finding is congruent with the findings of Mazis et al (1978).

In all, the study offers no answers but raises some interesting questions.

CRITICISMS

The study was flawed in that it evidently did not measure one or more important aspects of the literature's acceptability. Homogeneity of data suggests the questionnaire was insufficiently sensitive to indicate differences between groups. The sample used was big enough to be statistically viable for the tests utilized and those tests were appropriate to the data. The study population was small (n = 27) and it is possible a larger sample may elicit a difference not evident from this study. It is possible that patients would have been more critical in their appraisal of the materials offered them had they been given both texts and asked for comparative comments. These data could have been analysed using a t-test for matched samples (as opposed to unmatched samples) in much the same way. This method would have made it clearer to respondents that less favourable comments were acceptable. Obviously questions would have to be reworded. It is possible that this simple change may have made the findings rather more definitive.

IMPLICATIONS FOR FUTURE RESEARCH

This study has few direct implications for practice. Nonethelesss, as has been stated above, it raises some interesting questions and highlights the potential for future research both in terms of approach and subject matter.

Future quantitative approaches could, possibly, use the Cloze test. However, a research model utilizing a qualitative approach, perhaps grounded theory, might elicit hidden significances to which quantitative methods may be blind. Such a qualitative method could be applied to the investigation of readability as defined in this study. A viable 'halfway house' approach would be the use of a questionnaire with open-ended rather than closed questions; recurrent themes in patient responses could then be identified. Such a study could be effectively triangulated with interviews.

Readability as a tool with which to target patient information may be an incomplete indicator as there is a possibility that comprehensibility is at least as important and is not synonymous. The influence of this aspect of literature is currently underinvestigated (at least, the literature search as conducted for this study suggests so) and would be worthy of study. The development of a reliable and valid tool for healthcare staff to use in targeting literature accurately to their patients would prove an invaluable aid in ensuring that patients reap the maximum benefit from the increasing volume of written health education literature to which they are exposed.

SUMMARY OF FINDINGS

1. Patients receive written information favourably.
2. Raising the readability index of text appears to enhance the degree to which literature is favourably received.
3. No statistically significant differences between responses to literature with Flesch Reading Ease Scores of 49 and 63 were elicited.
4. Nurses reported that patients who had received the text with a higher readability index were better informed than the other group.
5. Readability, as such, is possibly only one aspect of successful material with comprehensibility being, perhaps, at least as important.
6. Further research would be of value with potential for a wide variety of different and complementary approaches being possible.

REFERENCES

Bourke G, Daily L, McGilvray J 1985 Interpretation and uses of medical statistics, 3rd edn. Blackwell Scientific, London
Boyd M, Citro K 1983 Cardiac patient education literature: can patients read what we give them? Journal of Cardiac Rehabilitation 3: 513–516
Burns N, Grove S K 1987 The practice of nursing research. W B Saunders, Philadelphia

Bauman A, Smith N, Braithwaite C, Free A, Saunders A 1989 Asthma information: can it be understood? Health Education and Research 4(3): 377–382

Couchman W, Dawson J 1990 Nursing and health care research. Scutari, London

Duryee R 1992 The efficacy of inpatient education after myocardial infarction. Heart and Lung 21(3): 217–224

Esty A, Musseau A, Keehn L 1991 Comprehension levels of patients reading health information. Patient Education and Counselling 18: 165–169

Evanoski C 1990 Health education for patients with ventricular tachycardia: assessment of readability. Cardiovascular Nursing 4(2): 1–6

Flesch R 1948 A new readability yardstick. Journal of Applied Psychology 32: 221–232

Gauld V 1981 Written advice: compliance and recall. Journal of the Royal College of General Practitioners 553–556

Glaser B, Strauss A 1967 The discovery of grounded theory: strategies for qualitative research. Weidenfeld and Nicolson, London

Gunning R 1952 The technique of clear writing. McGraw-Hill, New York

Hayward J 1975 Information – a prescription against pain. RCN, London

Herbet M 1990 Planning a research project. Cassell, London

Holcomb C, Ellis J 1978 The Cloze procedure. Health Education November: 8–10

Hussey L, Gilliland K 1989 Compliance: low literacy and locus of control. Nurse Clinician North America 24: 605–611

Kasprisin D, Clough P, Perisho A 1992 To improve communication, cultivate your writing. MLO October: 54–55

Klingelhofer E, Gershwin M 1988 Asthma self-management programs: premises, not promises. Journal of Asthma 25: 89–101

Larson I, Schumacher H 1992 Comparison of literacy level of patients in a VA arthritis centre with the reading level required by educational materials. Arthritis Care and Research 5(1): 13–16

Ley P 1988 Communicating with patients. Chapman and Hall, London

Lindeman C 1988 Patient education. Annual Review of Nursing Research 6: 29–60

Luker K, Caress A 1989 Rethinking patient education. Journal of Advanced Nursing 14: 711–718

Luther C, Allensworth D 1986 Evaluating printed materials. Nurse Educator 11(2): 18–22

Mazis M, Morris L, Gordon E 1978 Patient attitudes about two forms of oral contraception advice. Medical Care 16: 1045–1054

McLaughlin G 1969 SMOG grading – a new readability formula. Journal of Reading 12: 639–646

Meade C, Byrd J 1989 Patient literacy and the readability of smoking education literature. American Journal of Public Health 79(2): 204–206

Meade C, Smith C 1991 Readability formulas: cautions and criteria. Patient Education and Counselling 17(2): 153–158

Meade C, Wittbrot R 1988 Computerised readability analysis of written materials. Computers in Nursing 6(1): 30–36

Meade C, Diekmann J, Thornhill D 1992 Readability of American Cancer Society patient education literature. Oncology Nursing Forum 19(1): 51–55

Merritt S, Gates M, Skiba K 1993 Readability levels of selected hypercholesterolemia patient education literature. Heart and Lung 22(5): 415–420

Morris L, Halperin J 1979 Effects of written drug information on patient knowledge and compliance: a literature review. American Journal of Public Health 69: 47–52

Morris L, Kanouse D 1980 Consumer reactions to differing amounts of drug information. Drug Intelligence and Clinical Pharmacy 14: 531–536

Noble C 1991 Are nurses good educators? Journal of Advanced Nursing 6: 1185–1189

Owen P, Porter K, Frost C, O'Hare E, Johnson E 1993a Determination of the readability of educational materials for patients with cardiac disease. Journal of Cardiopulmonary Rehabilitation 13: 20–24

Owen P, Johnson K, Frost C, Porter K, O'Hare E 1993b Reading readability and patient education materials. Cardiovascular Nursing 29(2): 9–13

Pozen M 1977 A nurse rehabilitator's impact on patients with myocardial infarction. Medical Care 15: 830–837

Rahe R, Scalzi C, Shine K 1975 A teaching evaluation questionnaire for post myocardial infarction patients. Heart and Lung 4: 759–766

Raleigh E, Odtohan B 1987 The effect of a cardiac teaching program on patient rehabilitation. Heart and Lung 16: 311–317

Rankin S 1984 15 problems in patient education and their solutions. Nursing 14(4): 846–853

Rimm A, Hartz A 1980 Basic biostatistics in medicine and epidemiology. Appleton Century Crofts, New York

Silver R 1991 Guidelines: better information literature for hospital patients. King's Fund, London

Spadero D 1983 Assessing readability of patient information materials. Pediatric Nursing July/August: 274–278

Stephens S 1992 Patient education materials: are they readable? Oncology Nursing Forum 19(1): 83–85

Streiff L 1986 Can clients understand our instructions? Image 18: 48–51

Visser A 1980 Effects of an information booklet on well-being of hospital patients. Patient Counselling and Health Education 51–63

Walsh K 1991 Patient education. Plastic Surgical Nursing 11(3): 119–121

Young L, Humphrey M 1985 Cognitive methods of preparing women for hysterectomy: does a booklet help? British Journal of Clinical Psychology 24: 303–304

FURTHER READING

Cohen L, Manion L 1985 Research methods in education, 2nd edn. Croom Helm, Beckenham

Darling V, Rogers J 1986 Research for practising nurses. Macmillan, Basingstoke

Leddy S, Pepper J 1989 Conceptual basis of professional nursing. J B Lippincott, London

Ley P, Spelman M 1967 Communicating with the patient. Staples Press, London

Linde B, Janz N 1979 Effects of a teaching program on knowledge and compliance of cardiac patients. Nursing Research 28: 282–287

Macleod Clark J, Hockey L 1989 Further research for nursing. Scutari, London

Penckofer S, Llewellyn J 1989 Adherence to risk factor instruction one year following coronary artery by-pass graft surgery. Journal of Cardiovascular Nursing 3: 10–24

Squyres W 1980 Patient education: an enquiry into the state of the art. Springer, New York

Steele J, Ruzicki D 1987 An evaluation of the effectiveness of cardiac teaching during hospitalisation. Heart and Lung 16: 306–311

Treece E, Treece J 1986 Elements of research in nursing, 4th edn. C V Mosby, St Louis

Weinman J 1990 Providing written information for patients: psychological considerations. Journal of the Royal Society of Medicine 83: 303–305

Woods N, Catanzaro M 1988 Nursing research: theory and practice. C V Mosby, St Louis

Youngman M 1978 Designing and analysing questionnaires. Rediguide 12, TRC, Oxford

Patients' and nurses' experiences of feeding: a phenomenological study

Jan Dewing

Commentary

There was something that we both found very exciting about this chapter, which was initially constructed in part fulfillment of the requirements of a Masters in Nursing degree. It is presented here in a slightly annotated but still very detailed form.

In choosing feeding, Jan Dewing identified an area that is central and critical, and that may appear to encompass everything that is fundamental in good nursing practice, such as an awareness of physical and social needs, communication, the preservation of dignity, nurturance, 'being with' and caring. Despite this, despite feeding being one of the oldest, if not the oldest of all professional and non-professional nursing interventions, Jan's detailed literature review revealed that feeding is an area that has received practically no attention from nurse researchers. There are some exceptions of course, particularly the work of the Swedish nurse Norberg and her colleagues, some anecdotal accounts and the exploration of nutrition from various perspectives.

Jan appears to be the first to choose to explore the feelings of those being fed and of those doing the feeding. This was achieved by taking a phenomenological perspective and, as will be seen by reading the findings and discussion section, revealed a whole new world of feeding experiences, maintaining a high degree of truth value. The study that was produced is one that we are convinced carries considerable significance for the development of nursing practice and in particular in this, perhaps one of the most intimate aspects of nursing that can be performed.

Much is revealed by reading *Patients' and Nurses' Experiences of Feeding*. Firstly, the topic chosen is central to nursing practice yet it is a unique and innovative area of exploration. Secondly, the literature review is well constructed and the methodology succinctly described. Thirdly, the results are written up in such a style that it retains a high degree of truth value, in other words a 'yes I can identify with that' feel. All in all, the stuff of *real* nursing research!

ABSTRACT

Sometime after I started working in a unit for adults with physical disabilities I first became critically aware that I was not particularly knowledgeable and skilled at feeding patients. As I recall, I was talking with a group of patients about the presentation of meals following a report to me from the nurses that the food trolley was arriving with spilt food. The patients did not seem concerned about this issue but in the course of our conversation it became evident that they had views on other issues surrounding mealtimes and the food they were served. They described to me many issues which affected some or all of them. These included the way in which the dining area was arranged, the lack of choice about where they sat and who they had sitting next to them. Some patients mentioned the lack of privacy for eating as staff stood around the edges of the dining area and how this made them feel. These were only some of the issues we talked about. One patient said to me that he was not confident that the nurses knew how to feed him properly. He worried that when his voice and communication abilities deteriorated he may not be fed safely. He asked me to think about how that would feel to me.

I began to focus on my nursing skills with this aspect of my work with patients. I critically considered what I had done in my previous jobs and became aware that in most instances I had not developed positive strategies and interventions for feeding patients. I recollected patients that were 'difficult to feed'. I knew that I could not have described with any consistency or from any knowledge base my reasoning, decision making and action processes. Through observing and talking with my other nursing colleagues I became aware that they too had the same or similar difficulties. The more I reflected on the subject and the more I observed patients and nurses, the more complicated the subject became. This is how I became interested in patients' and nurses' experiences of feeding.

LITERATURE REVIEW

Introduction

Feeding, although a subject worthy of review in its own right, touches on several interrelated topics which were considered during the literature review. For purposes of order and clarity the original literature review was divided into seven sections, beginning with nutrition, then mealtimes, followed by sections on nursing skills, the nurse–patient relationship and patient ability, then a section on the environment and a final section that summarized the findings of the literature review. In this abridged version the first section on nutrition has been omitted and the remaining sections have been further edited.

The role of nurses in encouraging patients to eat, assisting patients to eat and teaching and supporting carers/relatives and other nursing staff in patient feeding is given minimal attention in most textbooks relating to the nursing care of adults. The text-book literature, for example, made statements that indicate nurses *should* encourage patients to eat and drink but the specific nursing strategies and their interventions are not considered. This was most obviously the case in the major nursing textbooks such as Judd (1983), Pritchard & Mallett (1992) and Royle & Walsh (1992). They were almost devoid of information on what to do with patients who need to be fed orally.

The absence of information could be for several reasons. Encouraging and assisting patients to eat is considered something that everyone, including nurses, can do. It is not considered to be a skilled activity or an important activity compared to some other nursing activities. Assisting people to eat must also compete with other tasks of a more technological and glamorous nature. Feeding people can be messy and time-consuming work but although a non-technological activity, it is still one that requires knowledge and competence to carry out effectively. There is mounting evidence to suggest that encouraging and assisting patients to eat and drink is a very complex and skilled activity involving a range of interrelated skills and interventions (Athlin & Norberg 1987, Norberg et al 1988).

Secondly, judging by the order in which information was presented and the amount of space occupied in articles and books, the authors of the literature reviewed appeared to regard technological intervention, such as dietary supplements and nasogastric/fine-bore tube feeding, as being more valuable than increasing the level of nursing intervention by feeding patients orally.

Thirdly, as the strategies and interventions involved in encouraging and assisting someone to eat are not clearly documented, it could be assumed that they have not been adequately explored and researched. There is an urgent need to ask how nurses learn to become competent in feeding patients and this could be an area for research in the future. However, progress in this field is unlikely whilst there is still interprofessional uncertainty about who exactly is responsible for the food intake, when patients need assistance.

Some authors, for example Gaskill & Pearson (1992), King et al

(1986) and Buergel (1979), identify the most appropriate person responsible for food intake as being the dietician. Other authors, whilst identifying the role of the dietician, more clearly indicate that nurses play an important role in providing nutritional support measures for patients (Williams & Copp 1990). Carr & Mitchell (1991) state that nurses are responsible for ensuring patients receive and eat their meals although many different personnel are likely to be involved in the provision of nutritional care. It has been suggested that serving meals is not a nursing responsibility (Tredger 1982) and in fact many meal delivery systems, ward layouts and rigid interpretation of Health & Safety regulations now ensure that the responsibility is taken away from nurses (Carr & Mitchell 1991). The type of involvement nurses have with patients and food should not be an either/or scenario. Both are extremes and lead to rigidity in practice and the establishment of routinized and ritualistic procedures. Nursing practice must be influenced by many factors, such as the reason for admission, the anticipated and actual length of stay, complications related to the illness, pathology, varying or changed patient ability and the catering and ward support services available and their flexibility.

Mealtimes in hospital

The literature connected with mealtimes seemed to concentrate on the role and activities of nurses around mealtimes (Carr & Mitchell 1991, Coates 1985) and the ability of nurses to accurately estimate the nutritional intake of patients during meals (Gaskill & Pearson 1992). The study by Gaskill & Pearson (1992) sought to explore the relationship between nurses' perception of dietary intake in a group of nutritionally vulnerable patients and their actual intake. Important inferences can be made from this study about the activities of nurses during mealtimes. The researchers intended to ask nurses to complete a record of dietary intake for each patient's meal. However, it proved impossible for this to be carried out. The nurses were only able to determine the patient's intake by what was served to them at the beginning of the meal. It can be inferred that the nurses were not directly involved in patients' mealtimes on a regular basis. The findings of the study highlighted that nurses either overestimated food intake or did not know the intake. As the authors indicated, this can mean delays in identifying malnourished patients. Although not identified by Gaskill & Pearson, it also means patients may experience hunger and thirst which can cause discomfort and distress.

Coates (1985 p 65) found that on two out of the three wards

she studied, nurses did supervise meals being given out but domestic staff cleared away trays at the end of meals. On the third ward only 46% of meals were supervised by nurses during the total observation period. Coates also found that nurses interrupted patients' mealtimes for the giving of medicines and even to perform pressure area care (p 77). This indicated that nurses gave a higher priority to their activities than to the patient-centred activity of mealtimes. The nurses may not have regarded meals as an event with any meaning in wider emotional, social and cultural terms but simply as the physical activity of eating food.

A study by Carr & Mitchell (1991) examined the care given to patients on medical wards during mealtimes. The researchers used two wards, one of which used food preplated in the main hospital kitchen (ward 1) and the other ward in which nurses served the food directly to patients (ward 2). The findings of the study indicated that nurses in ward 1 tended to be less involved with supervision of the meal trolley than nurses in ward 2. In this ward nurses were involved in the supervision of the meal trolley for 15 out of 22 meal observations (68.2%) which was three times more than the nurses on ward 1 (22.2% or four out of 18 observations). Nurses on both wards were not consistently involved in serving of meals although nurses on ward 2 directly served meals nine times (40.9%) compared with four times (22.2%) on ward 1.

Carr & Mitchell claimed that in theory, nurses who are supervising the serving of food are more likely to be involved in other aspects of mealtime care. This does not seem to have been the case in their study but the small size of the study makes any generalization unwise. This was a fact recognized by the authors themselves. Unfortunately, they do not clearly define what they meant by mealtime care. They talked about 'the patients' meal-related needs and specific feeding difficulties' but do not clarify their understanding of what constitutes either of these. This makes it impossible to evaluate the types of care given and the usefulness of them. This study seems to be primarily concerned with whether or not nurses initiated mealtime care and recognized feeding difficulties in patients. The authors did not look at what interventions were carried out by the nurses, the quality of the interventions or the outcomes for patients. Carr & Mitchell did state that most feeding difficulties went unnoticed by nurses and where interventions were made, it was generally by unqualified staff.

Mealtimes have the potential to be important events in our everyday lives, yet there appears to be some doubt about this in some of the literature regarding the psychological, social and cultural significance of mealtimes during hospitalization. Pearson (1989 p 130) described 'family type' meals in one clinical environment.

Ott et al (1990) argued that mealtimes are an opportunity for socialization, care giving and cultural acceptance. The same authors (1991) also argued that socialization at mealtimes stimulated interest with eating. They describe how 'family-style' meals were used to overcome the disadvantages of institutional-style meals. The authors did not describe what they regarded as a family-style meal so it is not possible to know if, for example, they took a stereotypical white middle class approach to what constituted a family-style meal. By institutional-style meals, the authors meant meals that were taken by large groups of patients in open-plan dining halls/rooms where the food is brought to the patient already plated. In their study four patients were assessed for their feeding abilities using standardized tests and then given the appropriate level of interventions to assist them to improve their level of independence. Possible interventions included postural repositioning, assistance to use feeding aids and equipment, changing table settings and lighting and introducing restaurant serving arrangements rather than serving compartmentalized preplated meals. Assistance was given by a therapist and could be either verbal and/or physical help and support.

At one level this study is interesting because of the assumptions it makes about the importance of socialization at mealtimes, in particular the value of creating a social environment and how this could influence food intake. However, socialization at mealtimes is not clearly defined. It could be that any interaction such as eye contact or simple verbal interactions such as 'pass the salt please' is considered to be meaningful social interaction. Equally it could be argued that simple instructional statements are not quality social interactions.

The study, because of a preoccupation with quantitative methodology, does not give any details about the types of interactions that took place between the subjects and the subjects and the therapist other than the instructions given to the patients. Patients were scored before and during therapist intervention. It should also be remembered that only four patients were used in this study. The criteria used for scoring included such items as being able to use feeding utensils correctly so if a patient used a knife or a spoon instead of a fork to eat peas with they were given a negative score. The researchers appeared to be imposing absolute norms on the patients rather than looking at the degree of progress made by each patient within their own established norms.

There is one further point arising from this study that is relevant. If social interaction at mealtimes did revolve around simple instructions directly related to eating food then serving restaurant-style meals as opposed to preplated food will promote interaction between some patients, because they will have to interact to eat their food. It may also have the effect of increasing their self-esteem and sense of social belonging. However, those patients who have poor perceptual and social skills may not be served adequately by this style of meal with the possible outcomes being a decrease in social identity, self-esteem and nutritional status.

A study by Sandman & Norberg (1988) supported this assumption. These researchers found that less able patients ate less complete meals. For example, they would serve themselves porridge but no milk or they would not take bread or potatoes with their main meal. They also found that these patients took less fluids than other more able patients. It could be more appropriate to patients' needs to have a variety of approaches to mealtimes instead of having one approach with which all patients are expected to comply.

Several studies considered the influence of the nurse's presence during patients' meals. For example, Davies & Snaith (1980) carried out a study to observe the amount and type of interactions at mealtimes on two long-stay wards for the elderly in the same hospital. They found twice as many interactions occurred on ward B than ward A and the type of interactions varied between the two wards. The researchers used non-participant observation of one meal on each ward. Both researchers observed three consecutive 15-minute intervals and recorded all the social interactions between patients and staff. The researchers had a 77% agreement on interobserver reliability which they described as satisfactory. The disagreement that occurred was due to omissions rather than disagreement over observation. The researchers did not comment on their experience as observers, the fact that two researchers both made consistent omissions in their observations or the reliability of the method they were using considering they reported the 23% omission rate.

The results of the Davies & Snaith study indicate 127 observations of interaction between patients and nurses, of which 41 were on ward A and 86 on ward B. The researchers devised a system of 11 interaction categories following data analysis. The researchers claim that these categories are mutually exclusive but they do not give any indication on the degree of difficulty encountered in making data fit into a category. For example, in the category *neutral supervisory comment*, a comment by a nurse such as 'Finished?' could also come into the *denial of choice* category.

In another study, Sandman & Norberg (1988) analysed the inter-action and behaviour of five patients with Alzheimer's disease and found that patients interacted more when left to eat on their own. The more able patients took on quasi-carer roles for the less able patients but when joined by nursing staff the inter-action became less and the carer-patients stopped their helping behaviours. The nurses' presence did mean that the less able patients ate more complete meals but providing the nutritional intake was already reasonable, it may have been more beneficial for the patients to be left on their own to interact with others. Learning or relearning social skills could lead to an increased food intake. It would appear from this study that nurses need to be aware of the effects of their presence during mealtimes with a social component. This study could also demonstrate the need for nurses to make more therapeutic use of the self when working with patients at mealtimes. None of the studies in this section provided any insight into what the nurses did and said with patients so no evaluation of their nursing skills was possible.

It would seem that mealtimes are significant events for patients but that the significance, especially from the social perspective, is not the same for all patients. Therefore shared mealtimes for all patients may not be suitable and although some healthcare professionals may introduce family-style dining experiences for patients it may not be suitable for all patients and may negatively influence their nutritional intake and other emotional and social skills. Furthermore, nurses appear to be unaware of how their presence and behaviours can influence patients' perceptions of their meals and perhaps their level of ability to eat independently for part of or all of a meal.

Nursing skills

It proved very difficult to find specific literature on nursing skills and feeding patients. This would seem to be at the core of what feeding patients is about from the nursing perspective and yet it is clearly missing from the literature. One particular researcher, Astrid Norberg, has contributed some useful research and much of her work will be considered in this section. It needs to be remembered that the work of Norberg and her colleagues was mostly carried out in Scandinavian countries and before any comparisons and generalizations can be made with our country, cultural factors need to be considered. For example, it may be that there are more or less positive attitudes to caring for elderly and disabled people in Scandinavian society. There may be more or less positive attitudes in the health and social services to working in elderly care institutions.

Assisting patients to eat and drink is not always a straight-forward activity in practice. In some cases giving food and drink to patients can cause discomfort and distress and yet as Norberg et al (1987a) comment, having food and drink withdrawn or withheld in any way can also cause discomfort and distress and eventually lead to death. This can affect both the patient and the nurse (Athlin & Norberg 1987).

Nurses can provide all the correct nutritional requirements for patients in attractive and socially and culturally acceptable presentations and yet patients can react in a variety of ways (Watson 1990). This can include refusal to eat the food and at the same time refusal to accept assistance. With some patients their response and behaviour with food is not constant. Norberg et al (1988) found that the feeding abilities of patients with Parkinson's disease and severe dementia varied over time. One of the patient participants in this study indicated that his abilities can change within the space of the same meal. Davies & Snaith (1980), as referred to in the previous section, found that although some patients were being fed by nurses they could assist themselves to feed for part of a meal even if it meant picking up food with their fingers. It is interesting to note that in one of the two wards they studied (ward A) nurses reprimanded patients for trying to feed themselves when the nurse was feeding them. Out of 13 observations coded in the category *denial of choice*, 11 were of this nature. This may again be an example of the professionals im-posing absolute norms on patients rather than facilitating patients to eat as best they can within their own norms and abilities even if it is only for part of a meal.

Norberg et al (1988), in a study involving 143 nursing assis-tants and 48 enrolled nurses in 23 nursing homes, attempted to find out how nursing staff perceived food refusal behaviours by patients and how they managed the patients when this behav-iour occurred. Semistructured interviews were carried out whilst being video recorded. In several of her studies Norberg uses video for recording interviews but does not give the rationale for using it; neither does she comment on how subjects may have been affected by the presence of a video but it can be assumed that the use of video enabled more than one researcher to analyse and categorize the data, therefore improving the reliability and validity of the findings.

The findings of this study revealed that 72.3% of nursing staff were able to provide accounts of patients who had refused to eat. This would have implications for the ways in which these nurses were prepared for assessing and carrying out interventions to cope with this type of patient behaviour. The researchers do not give any indication of whether the number of encounters provided by nursing staff were current or over a time span and if so what the time span was, so generalization is not advisable, although interviews were carried out over a period of 1 month. The researchers concluded that nursing staff were unable to differentiate between patients who refused food because of an apparent wish not to eat and those who refused food because they had lost the ability to eat. Furthermore, it appeared from the interviews that nursing staff responded with the same types of interventions for all patients who refused food, regardless of the reason for refusal. These interventions were aimed at making the patient eat rather than finding out the actual cause of the behaviour using assessment strategies to enable differentiation between patients who had lost the ability to eat and those who had not but were using food refusal behaviours.

At this point it is useful to make a distinction between refusing to eat and food-refusing behaviours. Norberg et al (1988) begin to suggest that there is a difference. Patients may refuse to eat because they have lost the ability to eat food, due to disease and impairment. Patients may use food refusal behaviours because they do not wish to eat, rather than being physically unable to do so. Food refusal behaviours may be present for other reasons, such as dislike of the food, the mealtime arrangements, dislike of the nursing staff feeding them, the way they are being fed or because of something that has previously affected the patient totally unconnected with the actual meal. The latter examples show how the use and abuse of food can give patients power over nurses and other carers. If nursing staff are unaware of the rationale for patients' behaviour and they react by trying to make the patient eat, mealtimes can be very stressful events as they become power struggles. Equally, nurses may too easily walk away from patients who may really want food but are unable to eat or even communicate their needs clearly. A review of the major clinical nursing textbooks, such as Perry & Potter (1990), Pritchard & Mallett (1992) and Royle & Walsh (1992), indicated that differentiation in the assessment of eating abilities is not considered and in most of the text books no assessment of food-refusing behaviour is considered. Backstrom et al (1987) suggested that nursing staff did not feed the same patients regularly as a means of limiting the stressful effects of patients refusing food. It would appear that the nurses found feeding patients a stressful activity. Furthermore, it suggests that nursing skills were lacking and the way that nurses acted maintained the situation rather than managed it. Rather than identifying the real reasons patients are refusing food, nurses contained their stress by avoidance techniques.

Other studies have considered the way in which nursing work is organized and whether or not this influences nursing skills in feeding patients. Athlin & Norberg (1987) suggested that attitudes to and interpretations of the behaviours by patients during feeding are more positive with a patient allocation system of nursing than in a task allocation system. They devised a study involving six patients and four nurses, where the same nurse fed the same patient for 14 consecutive meals, over several spans of duty. The researchers interviewed the nurses after meals 1, 7 and 14. The researchers described how the organization of the meals on the ward was changed from task allocation to patient allocation. They do not indicate if this was a change they engineered for the purposes of the study and they do not indicate how the nurses were prepared for the change. Neither do they say if the change was for all patients or only the four patients included in the study. The change also only seems to be for mealtime care and not for all patient care, thus calling into doubt the organization of care. The qualitative data analysis seems to indicate that the nurses did have more positive attitudes not only to feeding the patients but also to the patients themselves. However, this was not the case for all the nurses involved in the study.

Athlin & Norberg (1987) concluded that patient allocation was a more beneficial system of nursing for feeding patients with difficult eating behaviours and altered feeding abilities. The researchers referred to the work of Scheflin on the signal model of interaction (Scheflin 1975). They suggested that because communication can become a problem in many patients who need feeding, this model is useful for nursing when used with a patient allocation system. The model itself does not emphasize that where patients can no longer clearly communicate using language and gestures, the nurse and patient need to establish an alternative system of communication that relies on more subtle cues and interpretations. A major flaw in the construction of the link between the signal model and patient allocation is that changing to patient allocation does not necessarily improve the sensitivity or skills of nurses, it may simply involve an organizational change.

However, it may enable nurses to practise more effectively if they have good communication skills already. Nurses must have the skills or the awareness to cue into the patients' behaviour in the first place.

Most of the research on non-verbal interaction during assisted feeding has been done with infants, children (disabled and able-bodied) and their main caregiver, generally their mother. The description of such feeding by Barnard (1981) is used by Norberg & Athlin (1987) as the basis for a model for the assessment of interaction between patients with Parkinson's disease and their caregivers during assisted feeding. At the centre of this model lie the features of interaction between the patient and the caregiver: clarity of cues, sensitivity, interpretation and responsiveness with the aim of achieving synchronicity between the two individuals. This appears to complement the signal model approach although it is more sophisticated. The degree of success of the interaction is partly dependent on the caregiver's level of empathy with the patient. It must be recognized that several external variables still influence the success of interactions, including the organization of nursing, the philosophy of nursing and educational input into the area.

At one level this model is useful for practice because it focuses the concerns of the nurse on the patient's perspective. It also enables nurses to think about achieving synchronicity with the patient. This can be likened to artistic movement and dance. Gendron (1988 p 24) likened synchronous interaction to orchestral music and argued it is related to feelings of well-being. Both the nurse and patient need to communicate, even if words are not always used. They need to achieve a flowing exchange that enables each person to achieve their aims but also enables the other person to do the same. Achieving synchronicity occurs in different ways. For some patients it is ongoing during the meal, balancing the task of feeding with the emotional and social aspects of care during feeding. From the literature it can be seen that patients with Parkinson's disease cannot always focus on socioemotional activities at the same time as being assisted to eat or trying to eat independently. Assisted feeding with these patients must concentrate on the task, with the nurse acting as an instrument for the patient's feeding (Norberg & Athlin 1987). This does not mean socioemotional needs are not included in mealtime care. The nurse must plan to meet these needs before and after the task of feeding. The interaction model, although useful, leaves too many unanswered assumptions, especially concerning the influences of the external variables on the actual nurse–patient interaction, such as the effect of the environment or the nurse's levels of knowledge and skills.

In a study looking at the effect of educational input on feeding, Kolodny & Malek (1991) found that following educational input from expert professionals, nurses still continued to feed patients inconsistently and in an unsafe manner. This may say more about the inappropriateness of the educational input than the nursing skills. Unfortunately the author does not indicate what the programme involved, how detailed it was or how practice specific it was.

As a result of reviewing the literature in this section it can be concluded that there was very little literature specifically related to the skills nurses need to use to feed patients in patient-centred ways or much evidence of good practice that nurses were doing this. There was a distinct lack of information in the major nursing textbooks about feeding and this is more marked when the amount of information about other nursing activities or patients' needs, such as elimination and continence, are compared with the amount of literature available on feeding. Assisting patients to eat is influenced by several interdependent factors at different levels, including the skills of nurses to communicate meaningfully with patients and enable the patient to communicate with them as a part of the feeding experience. Nurses need to harmonize effective forms of communication with the actual task of feeding to achieve a kind of synchronicity. It would appear that nurses regard feeding as primarily a task and one that has not been incorporated into individualized patient care systems. This may be due to nursing preferences as the literature has indicated nurses seemed to find feeding patients a difficult and personally stressful task/activity and therefore seek to avoid it, although this practice may not be in the best interests of patients.

Nurse–patient relationships

Feeding another person is an intimate personal activity, which not only involves doing a task but involves a set of communication issues as demonstrated in the last section and as such its significance needs to be considered within the relationships of the people involved (Norberg et al 1980). Norberg et al (1987a) suggest that the withdrawal or withholding of food and fluid from certain patients can imply that they are regarded as less valuable than other persons. This demonstrates how nurses can use food as a means of power over patients. Food does not always need to be withdrawn or withheld; demonstration of power may involve giving a different type and quality of food to one patient as opposed to others or making patients wait, for example. The literature contains examples of some of the problematic areas associated with feeding patients: for example, patients being arranged in certain seating positions to enable staff to feed more than one patient at the same time (Ott et al 1991), infusing and tube feeding dying patients (Norberg et al 1980). Forceful feeding of patients is another problem area. Norberg et al (1988) described how nursing staff would use a range of feeding techniques including opening patients' mouths with spoons or their fingers or gripping the patient's nostrils in order to make the patient open their mouth.

Kolodny & Malek (1991) described only in general terms how nurses fed patients in a way that did not always ensure a safe and dignified experience for patients. Athlin & Norberg (1987) found that the nurses in their study often expressed anxiety or fear about feeding patients who they described as difficult to feed. Norberg et al (1980) concluded that the failure of nurses to understand the behaviour of dying patients led to conflict and anxiety in the nurses and the patients. In turn this resulted in the setting up of infusions and tube feeding, etc., essentially to relieve the nurses' anxiety rather than always acting in the best interests of the patients.

In the literature reviewed it was not possible to find anything close to a framework accounting for the reasons why patients refuse to eat or to be fed and this is clearly an area for future research, although a sensitive and challenging one. The literature, especially in the major nursing textbooks, did make reference to physiological problems such as disease, lack of appetite and poorly fitting dentures (Axelsson et al 1984, Middleton 1983, Perry & Potter 1990). It is not surprising that nurses become anxious about what to do when they encounter problems with feeding in their practice, especially when it becomes obvious that the transitions from accepting food, eating and accepting feeding to refusing food, refusing to eat and refusing to be fed are not clearly described in nursing literature. Patients' behaviour may have different meanings which must be interpreted correctly. To do this the nurses need to have close relationships with patients. In part this is influenced by the organization of nursing on the ward, having a nursing philosophy that expresses a belief in individualized care and the operationalization of that philosophy. Even with individualized patient care systems nurses did not necessarily see feeding patients as part of a whole relationship they had with the patient, as some of the data in this study have identified.

Nurses need to understand that patients can choose to use feeding as a means of exerting control over their life and over the people around them, no matter how ill they may be. Patients can choose to use feeding as a means of having more or less nursing contact around them. As Norberg et al (1980) comment, if the quality of the contact with the nurses is not what is wanted by the patient they may become even less satisfied and escalate food-refusing or abusing behaviour. Equally, the same authors comment that patients who are dying can control their fluid intake to influence the level of anxiety in nurses, thus achieving control over the nurses and death to a certain extent and for a certain length of time. In practice situations, nurses would tend to react negatively to these types of scenarios and may not have interpreted patient behaviours correctly.

The same authors describe three possible sets of conflicts in situations where patients refuse or are unable to accept feeding. Firstly, there is a conflict between the nurse's responsibility to feed the patient and the patient's refusal to be fed. Secondly, a conflict exists between the nurse's duty to keep the patient alive but not to make the patient experience prolonged suffering and finally there is a conflict between the inevitability of death and the nurse's or patient's reluctance to accept death as an outcome. The authors conclude that this effectively sets up a double-bind situation so that whatever action the nurse takes can be perceived as being wrong.

Backstrom et al (1987), in a study examining feeding difficulties in long-stay patients, found that only 14 patients out of 113 had the same caregiver to feed them for two or three consecutive meals. Additionally they found that many patients had 16–20 different caregivers feeding them during the observation period of 28 days, with a maximum of 30 different caregivers. Norberg et al (1988) similarly found that the median number of nursing staff feeding each patient during the same time period was 18. In the 1987 study the researchers asked caregivers to make notes about feeding difficulties experienced by patients during every meal over a 28-day span. Most caregivers gave very limited comments on patients' difficulties with feeding, which were described by caregivers as 'just the same as always'. Caregivers gave such comments because they hardly knew the patients they were feeding. The caregivers, in order to provide such comments, must have been comparing each patient with another patient or with some idea in their own mind rather than comparing each patient with their own norm. They appeared unable to provide patient-centred comments because they did not establish regular contact with patients for feeding. It could also be argued that they perceived feeding as a task rather than a patient and nurse activity. The researchers concluded by stating that 'a system of task allocation could not create situations which promote self-feeding or harmonious assisted feeding' (Backstrom et al 1987).

A similar conclusion was made in a study by Athlin & Norberg (1987) who went on to suggest that patient allocation systems such as primary nursing facilitated the development of more personalized nurse–patient relationships which is beneficial for the nurse and patient when it involves feeding. But it must be said that there is no conclusive evidence to suggest that this was actually the case. The introduction of primary nursing systems would not necessarily change nurse knowledge and skills in areas associated with feeding.

There is some positive evidence in the literature about the benefits of individualized patient care systems. Norberg et al (1988) suggested that nursing organized around individualized patient care enabled nursing staff to feel more certain about how to interpret patients' feeding behaviours and how to deal with them. The researchers used findings from another study (Athlin & Norberg 1987) to validate their comments. Because Norberg and her colleagues have carried out much of the research into patient feeding they tend to constantly refer to their own previous work. This is legitimate if the previous work is reputable. In this particular instance the researchers made unreasonable comments about the benefits of individualized patient care. Nurses need to have an intimate relationship with patients who require feeding and especially with patients who are difficult to feed for whatever reasons. However, this alone is insufficient and nurses clearly require skilful feeding techniques and an understanding of the overall situation in order to be able to interpret patient behaviour accurately.

This section has further highlighted the interdependency between the factors at different levels that can influence the experience of feeding for patients and nurses. Patients who have complex feeding requirements or who are at transition phases, for example between accepting assistance with feeding and refusing assistance, caused nurses great concern. The literature indicated that nurses did not fully understand the behaviour of patients in the context of how they used food as a form of control or as an emotional, social or cultural statement. It would appear from the literature reviewed that nurses did not have a range of skills to use in these situations but it would also seem that when nurses did try to carry out interventions they were often in a double-bind where there was a no-win situation for both the nurses and the patients.

Patient ability

The ageing process includes physical, sensory and perceptual changes that can affect elderly people's motivation and ability to eat and to feed themselves independently (Ott et al 1991). Eating problems are also associated with some diseases such as cerebrovascular accidents, Parkinson's disease, arthritis and multiple sclerosis. In a study by Backstrom et al (1987), of 214 patients observed 110 patients had eating problems from dementia, 30 from cerebrovascular accidents and 16 as a result of Parkinson's disease. The other patients were not described.

In another study by Sandman et al (1990), it was found that out of 3607 patients in elderly long-term care placements, 10% were dependent for feeding. The researchers also found that loss of ability to eat was related to an inability to perform other activities of daily living. They supported the hypothesis of Katz et al (1963, cited in Katz & Akpom 1976) that feeding is a simple motor and neurological function compared with, for example, dressing which is a complex function. For Katz et al, the significance of this was that complex functions regress first and simple functions last, in the reverse order of child development.

In view of the information gained through this review it does not seem appropriate to regard feeding as a simple motor activity. Katz et al were looking at feeding in the context of the medical model and therefore with a physiological bias as well. The findings of Katz et al may be true with elderly people but as Sandman et al (1990) indicated, their conclusion is still questionable. Katz et al made no attempt to differentiate between inability to eat and food-refusing behaviour which may appear as an inability to eat. What the researchers did find, which supports the findings by Katz et al, was that 98% of those patients dependent for feeding were also dependent for continence needs, mobility (95%) and washing and dressing (99%). As 84% of the patients with these dependencies had a diagnosis of dementia it should be pointed out that the researchers may have had difficulty in clearly assessing levels of ability in daily activity as the cooperation and ability levels of the patients may have varied. The researchers did make use of various tools for assessments but did not comment on any methodological issues that may have arisen from the use of the tools.

It has been suggested that as part of a universal ageing process elderly people gradually disengage from society (Cumming & Henry 1961). However, as Davies & Snaith (1980) argued, it is more likely that society disengages from the elderly. In terms of elderly or disabled people being patients, it could be that nurses and patients have certain preconceptions about what abilities patients should have. It may be acceptable to need care and therapy for mobility and continence needs but not to need feeding. To require assistance with eating may be viewed by many healthcare workers as being an additional requirement for care rather than part of daily needs.

Much of the literature indicated nurses have negative attitudes to feeding. The term 'feeding' itself holds negative connotations. It suggests a picture of someone who is infantile and dependent whereas the term 'assisted eating' or 'assistance with eating' sounds much more positive and respectful of the individual's dignity. Feeding is an activity associated with babies and infants. Given that feeding patients is a complex aspect of nursing care, the literature should contain information on how to improve patients' eating and feeding skills so that they remain as independent as they possibly can, but this is not the case. The major nursing textbooks contain little useful information on promoting independent eating skills and neither do they adequately cover assessment of patient abilities. Some of the literature in this review has indicated nurses tended to discourage patients from feeding themselves some parts of a meal when the nurses perceived they needed nursing assistance (Sandman & Norberg 1988).

Axelsson et al (1984) found that the length of stay in hospital for patients with eating problems following a stroke was greater than those without eating problems, on average by 22 days. They also found that patients requiring long-term care were more likely to need feeding than those who did not have long-term care. This may give an indication of the level of social acceptability concerned with feeding, that patients who needed feeding were more likely to be cared for in an institution than at home in the community. By using observational assessment techniques these researchers were able to demonstrate the exact problems with eating in stroke patients; 46 patients were observed and it was found that each patient had more than one problem. Some of the problems included hoarding food in the mouth (33 patients), leakage of food from the mouth (31 patients) and chewing problems (31 patients). It may be possible that some difficulties with feeding existed prior to the stroke. These are all problems that could be regarded as socially unacceptable. But as Axelsson et al (1986) demonstrated, it is possible to correct these problems where a patient-centred rehabilitation programme for relearning eating skills is used.

As a result of this research, the authors suggested a model of the factors influencing eating problems in patients with a stroke. The components of the model involve prestroke physical state, physical consequences of eating problems, neurological deficits, psychological factors and social and cultural factors. Through the expanded discussion of how the model can be used it was made clear that each of the components is multifacetted and inter-dependent with the other components in the model. The authors stated that the model is simplistic but it does at least begin to provide a framework that clinical nurses could use when working with patients who have experienced eating problems through a stroke. I would argue that using such a model would require nurses to assess patient needs and abilities, which would mean longer periods of contact with patients than would be involved in a task approach to mealtimes and feeding. This argument supports those of Athlin & Norberg (1987) and Backstrom et al (1987) who argue for individualized patient care systems.

A more detailed model has been suggested for the assessment of eating problems in patients with Parkinson's disease (Norberg et al 1987b). The authors produced the model as a result of ex-tensive literature reviews rather than actual research. They also drew from literature that used brain-damaged animals in their research. Therefore great caution must be made when applying any of the findings from this type of research to humans.

The model starts by using the World Health Organization's classification of impairment, disability and handicap. This, it could be argued, is a fundamental flaw in the model because the classi-fication assumes a causal sequence to impairment, disability and handicap, thus giving the model a reductionist approach as some eating problems (i.e. food-refusing behaviours) may not be di-rectly connected with disease. In the part of the model looking at handicap, Erikson's theory of the eight stages of man is used (Erikson 1982). This provides a less reductionist but novel ap-proach to the model. It introduces nurses to the idea that patients constantly face dilemmas or crises if they experience difficulties in eating. During each crisis patients have to come to a solution from two opposing attitudes towards life. The authors provide a discussion of the possible opposing attitudes to life that can be faced by patients. An example of this is industry–inferiority (or incompetence). Patients have to decide between struggling to continue to eat independently despite the effort involved or feel-ing a loss of competence by asking for and receiving assistance.

The incorporation of Erikson's theory does offer the potential for nurses to try and understand what feeding means for patients and how the process of coming to recognize and accept or reject assistance with feeding is a complex series of crises for patients.

In another paper using Erikson's theory, a man with a stroke of 3 years' duration was reintroduced to solid food, having been supplied with a liquid diet via a nasogastric tube for 3 years (Axelsson et al 1986). This patient, when interviewed, described his main problems as having to eat in isolation from his family, craving for the sensation of food in his mouth and feeling depressed that he did not have a normal life without being able to eat food. Erikson's theory is almost incidental in the paper other than the researchers talking about aspects of trust–mistrust (hope) as the patient undergoes a programme of rehabilitation to relearn how to eat. But the paper is useful as a case study because it demonstrates specific aspects of nursing assessment and feeding skills, incorporating teaching, and this is described within the context of developing a relationship with the patient and the carer. It describes what can be achieved when nursing skills are used effectively.

An interesting observation is made by the researchers when they state that the patient's level of ability in other activities of living, namely washing, dressing and mobility, quickly improved once the patient began to eat without a nasogastric tube. It may be that achieving improved levels of independence in eating, particularly without external appliances such as tubes, is a significant factor in increasing hope and self-esteem. As described earlier, Katz et al (1963, cited in Katz & Akpom 1976) identified a relationship between feeding and the other activities of living. However, it may be that if nurses and other healthcare professionals focused more on enabling patients to eat as independently as possible, other activities of daily living could be improved as more motivation comes from the patients. The researchers concluded that an important aim of the programme was to assist the patient to gain insight into his own problems and not to be conditioned by healthcare professionals into a fixed level of ability and dependence. Finally, the researchers go on to say:

The nurse's most important task is to understand the patient's experiences and attitudes, to identify his reasons for mistrust and to remove or counterbalance them through teaching, training and support.

In summary, nurses appear not to accurately assess patients' abilities to eat independently. Patients with some conditions such as a stroke have specific difficulties in eating. These patients can be regarded negatively by nurses and perhaps by society. Patients with long-term feeding needs are more likely to be placed in institutional care settings than remain in the community. Patients who need feeding may stay in hospital longer than those who do not need feeding. Given these facts, nurses should be investing in assessment and rehabilitation programmes to assist patients to improve their feeding skills. The literature review has suggested two models that can be used for working with patients who need feeding. These models attempted to put the experience of feeding into patient-centred perspectives and into the context of considering the impact needing to be fed has on the patient's abilities and on their life and social roles.

The environment

There is evidence to suggest that some patients do respond to changes in the environment where feeding takes place (Ott et al 1990). Watson (1990) has reviewed some of the literature concerned with the effect of the environment on elderly people with dementia and concluded that improved decor, less institutional serving arrangements of food and altered seating patterns can all produce positive changes in patients' behaviour.

In a study by Deutekom et al (1991) patients were asked, using a crude 3-point scale, if a sociable atmosphere and a quiet environment for mealtimes were being provided. The authors describe these two variables as producing a sociable environment for mealtimes, although no clear description of what constitutes a sociable environment for mealtimes is provided. The authors wanted to find out if the nursing textbooks' prescription that a quiet relaxed environment should be provided during mealtimes was being carried out in practice. The findings of this study indicated that 5% of patients reported an unquiet atmosphere and 18% reported that the atmosphere in their room was not sociable during mealtimes. The researchers observed the interruptions made by nurses, other healthcare staff, visitors and support service staff such as housekeepers. Most interruptions were made by nurses (44%). This supports the findings by Coates (1985 p 77). Although Coates did not give any statistics she stated that nurses interrupted meals for medicine giving and sometimes to perform pressure area care.

However, in the Deutekom study the researchers who were directly observing mealtimes sat outside patients' rooms rather than in the rooms so they were unable to ascertain why the nurses interrupted patients' mealtimes and if the patients perceived all nursing activity as an interruption. It could be that the physical presence of the nurse did not actually disturb or stop the patient from eating. However, it can be inferred that some of the nurse interruptions were not directly connected with patients' meals and could have been avoided, as the findings indicated they were not related to other direct care needs.

It is interesting to note that 34% of the interruptions were made by therapists, doctors, visitors, housekeepers and social workers. This amount of interruption is significant when considered that these staff do not need to be involved in patients' mealtimes. Out of 86 observations only 17 patients had no interruptions for a period of 15 minutes or more. The authors' main finding was that the amount of food left on plates correlated with interruptions made by staff other than nurses. An interesting comment is made in relation to the effect other patients have on promoting a positive environment conducive to quiet and peaceful mealtimes. Deutekom et al state that patients could be requested to cooperate to some extent during mealtimes by staying near to their bed or table until other patients have finished their meals. Although the authors made no other comment, the possible effect of patients on each other at mealtimes was something that I decided to consider.

Ott et al (1990) documented their concern about the lack of social interaction at mealtimes amongst patients in a particular extended care unit. They undertook a literature review to assist them to improve mealtime functioning for the elderly residents. Providing a social environment may not agree with the findings of the study by Deutekom et al (1991) where it was concluded most patients want a quiet and peaceful environment. Additionally, findings by Norberg & Athlin (1987) indicate that patients with certain impairments need to be quiet and undisturbed by social tasks whilst eating. Beck (1981) found that those whom elderly people sit next to at mealtimes can determine the amount of food they eat and their enjoyment of the meal.

There is little literature on the effects patients have on each other during mealtimes. Although mealtimes have psychological, social and cultural significance, especially in our daily lives with families and friends, it may be that when patients are hospitalized or live in institutions, mealtimes become less significant. The efforts of healthcare professionals to create social interactions and a social atmosphere at mealtimes may not always be appropriate where patients have no choice about whom they share their meal with and whom they have to sit next to. It may be even less appropriate where, because of physical or mental impairment, patients need to concentrate on maintaining their independent feeding skills.

Summary

Eating and drinking have great social and cultural significance and for most healthy people are sources of great enjoyment. What we eat and how we eat are reflective of our abilities to function independently and as Glenn et al (1993) comment, restoring levels of independence in feeding following illness is essential to achieving an acceptable level of personal and social functioning. When significant impairment, either through disease and/or ageing and hospitalization exists, unique problems arise in the relationship between food, eating and nutritional status. There is evidence to suggest that the risk of malnutrition occurs proportionally to the length of time spent in hospital for all patients (Coates 1985 p 13). Therefore the risk for patients who are unable to eat or refuse food for whatever reasons must be significantly greater. There are several factors which influence the relationship between food, eating and nutritional status that have been critically reviewed as part of this dissertation. There is some evidence in the literature covering some of the areas of nursing practice although it generally tends to be more quantitative in nature and therefore looks at issues independently of each other. There is a need for further research to understand the social significance of mealtimes for people whilst in hospital and to evaluate the appropriateness of family or communal-style dining experiences.

The literature review has also identified the need to expand nursing knowledge about the ways in which food can be used as a form of control by nurses and patients.

The work by Norberg and her colleagues has provided much of the background reading for some sections of this literature review and it was one of her papers that originally led this researcher to take a more indepth look at the area of feeding in practice and now as a formal research study. Without the work of Norberg the nursing literature would be essentially devoid of current research into this area of nursing practice. This is surprising as for many nurses the activity of feeding patients, to one degree or another, must be a regular one. There is a mass of information in the literature, both journals and books, on other regular nursing activities such as dealing with the elimination and mobility needs of patients but not with feeding, although there is more information on meeting nutritional needs, an area associated with feeding.

The relationships between food, feeding, nurses and patients and the environment are some of the most important factors that can influence the experience of feeding and yet they are so clearly missing from the literature. An area of concern identified by this review is that the main nursing textbooks likely to be used by student and clinical nurses and available on ward libraries contain very little information about feeding patients and the nursing skills required to deal with patients who need feeding and those who refuse to eat and to be fed. Another area of concern is that the literature does not describe feeding from the perspective of patients. In all the research literature reviewed, only one paper was found that made any direct reference to how patients perceive difficulties in eating and being fed and even then it was incidental data (Axelsson et al 1986).

This literature review has found some research that gives useful insights into the experience of feeding but nothing that describes and gives meaning to the total experience of feeding for nurses and patients. No nursing literature similar to the area under study in this dissertation was found in the fairly extensive search carried out for this review. Research has focused on analysing what nurses seem to be doing by observing them from a distance or indirectly, rather than working with nurses to enable them to describe and come to understand how they are working with patients. The emphasis has been on building up only one part of the total picture. This research study and dissertation is therefore contributing to the very limited existing knowledge in the area of feeding.

METHODOLOGY

Introduction

A large amount of editing has taken place in this section as the original dissertation was prepared as part of the course requirements for a Masters in Nursing degree. This section on methodology originally contained a debate on the value of quantitative and qualitative research, issues in connection with choosing the most appropriate methodology and other related topics.

Selecting a qualitative methodology

Once I accepted that it was valid to use a qualitative approach and that this could be justified, it then became necessary to work through the mass of information about the different types of qualitative research methodologies to see exactly where this study belonged in the qualitative domain. At this stage the ideas about the study were still very basic. It was both appealing and yet an issue of concern that it would have been possible to make the study fit a methodology, just to give it a clear identity and structure. Swanson-Kauffman (1986) has commented that in qualitative research there seems to be a temptation to make studies fit clearly into one of the types or modes of qualitative research, perhaps in order to enable the researcher to argue with conviction that they are using accepted methods for their research.

The issue of identifying where in the qualitative domain the methodology belonged was not straightforward and uncomplicated. It may be that grasping qualitative methods was a more complex and demanding task, as Nieswiadomy (1987 p 48) commented can be the case. This serves to illustrate the usefulness of piloting methods before undertaking the main data collection. Piloting of the methods did take place in this study using one patient and one nurse participant. During the period of data collection the patient became acutely ill so the data were incomplete and not included in the study. The piloting did, however, act as a rehearsal for the live data collection. It allowed some modifications to take place that otherwise would have interfered with the main data collection.

Qualitative methodologies

Through a process of critical review it emerged that the methodology chosen for this research study most closely resembled phenomenology. A critical review of the value and relevance of three main qualitative methodologies was necessary to demonstrate their degree of appropriateness for this study. The methods that were considered were phenomenology, grounded theory and ethnography. This task was complicated by the fact that aspects of all three methodologies at some time seemed appropriate. For example, this study did involve some consideration of the social environment in which participants were being fed and how that environment influenced patients and nurses participating in the study, thus bringing into consideration an ethnographic approach. However, the influence of the environment had to be considered a part of the components that made up the total (or whole) experience of feeding for nurses and patients. The social environment could not be ignored but including it in the study did not make the study an ethnographic one. For this and many other reasons it was concluded that this study involves some blurring of methodological boundaries to incorporate ethnographic elements. This illustrated what Swanson-Kauffman (1986) described as the matrix formation of qualitative methodology.

This study was more concerned with the human experience of feeding than with looking at the relationship between themes and patterns concerned with feeding in the context of a cultural analysis of nursing, thus coming to the conclusion that the chosen methodology tends more towards phenomenology than ethnography.

Phenomenology

Essentially phenomenological research is about trying to describe lived experiences of those studied by the use of four basic strategies. These strategies are described by Swanson-Kauffman & Schonwald (1988 p 98) as bracketing, analysing, intuiting and describing. These authors go on to state that data are gathered, sorted, retrieved, condensed and verified (p 100). Bracketing is a particularly contentious issue and is considered in the section on ethics.

Phenomenology is a descriptive approach to research that has as its objective identifying human behaviour in order to promote an understanding of human behaviour as a whole. Generally phenomenology is not about interpreting data and applying alternative words or language to explain and account for the way experiences occur but it is about 'telling it as it is' (Field & Morse 1985 p 28). However, hermeneutics, a branch of phenomenology, does involve interpretative elements rather than description only (Reeder 1988 p 193).

In this study it could be argued that the questions used during interview were of a phenomenological nature. For example, the question 'Can you tell me what it's like to be fed?' was asked of all the patient participants in all the interviews, as was the question 'Can you tell me what it's like to feed this patient?' of all the nurse participants. This study had as its focus the lived experience of the participants, although it also considered the context or environment in which the events and interactions took place. This was felt to be important because patients were not in their usual roles or taking meals in their usual environment. After revisiting the literature review and reflecting on the questions that had originally generated interest in the issue of feeding, it became clearer that the central issue of what it is like to be fed and to feed required a phenomenological base. Furthermore, as the literature review established, there is little information about how feeding and being fed affect nurses and patients so carrying out research using a phenomenological approach was not unreasonable.

The intended and actual data analysis involved describing what was happening during feeding and mealtimes between nurses and patients. This was consistent with the phenomenological approach because the process of analysis aimed to maintain the essence of the data and to remain true to the experience as lived by the participants. During the initial analysis of data alternative words were used at times to describe the experience. This meant that interpretation had occurred and the reality of the actual experience had been changed. It was extremely difficult not to fall into interpretation; remaining consistently true to describing data is obviously a learned skill. It may also be that as nurses we have been used to interpreting what patients say into nursing or medical frameworks and models rather than accepting reality and meaning as the patient describes them. It is impossible not to interpret data, either as they are being collected or later for purposes of analysis.

The apparent need to have an officially sanctioned qualitative methodology caused much concern during the process of this research. Swanson-Kauffman (1986) appears to have experienced the same dilemma. This author stated that nurses should let the nursing questions guide the methods while being ever aware that the methods utilized will shape the answers. It requires some confidence and experience to ride this storm. Some qualitative research can involve a mixing of methods. Swanson-Kauffman (1986) described how in a particular study exploring the human experience of miscarriage, the methodology evolved into a unique blending of phenomenological, ethnographic and grounded theory methods. Morse (1991 pp 15 and 20) referred to this study and described this mixing as 'do-able' but claimed it violated epistemological assumptions of all the methods used. Thus it becomes bad science.

Morse is clearly stating that the utilization of qualitative methods is not just a case of selecting the most suitable method. Researchers must have an understanding of the theories and their assumptions that underpin the methodologies they choose to use. This is an important argument because the use of a particular methodology makes a statement about the type of knowledge that is valued by the researcher and the type of knowledge other members of nursing are gaining access and exposure to. However, this argument is still in the arena of choosing one mode over another. Although it is not saying 'choose between quantitative or qualitative' it is simply replacing that debate with a new one of choosing one qualitative method as being superior to another.

The new debate is of choosing between one or other of the qualitative modes as if they were in separate camps with definable boundaries. Therefore feminist researchers will always use feminist research methods and so on. Swanson & Chenitz (1982) more usefully regard different qualitative methodologies as being on a continuum rather than being in different camps. If the notion of the research methodologies being on a continuum is accepted then blurring should not be problematic. Thus there is some blurring of the methodology in this study. However, this is not to argue that the researcher has used a mixed method approach. There was no deliberate intention for a mixed method to be used. Nor is it to argue that in qualitative research mixing methods is bad science, as argued by Morse. Swanson-Kauffman (1986) referred to combined methods and not to mixed methods. The arguments of Swanson-Kauffman in support of combined methods are more reasonable.

In summary, phenomenology is not about building theories of nursing, although it may provide some concepts for theory building. Phenomenology is about trying to understand the lived experience of people (Anderson 1991 p 36, Lynch-Sauer 1985 p 93) and as such it was selected as being the most appropriate methodological approach for this study.

Phenomenological methodology and analysis must keep to the essence of the experience under study. Trying to work out the exact research mode this study belongs to has been extremely challenging. It is possible to say that this study very clearly involves a qualitative investigation. It met most of the 10 criteria identified by Cobb & Hagemaster (1987) to qualify as a qualitative research study. However, it is also possible to argue that whilst phenomenology is the most appropriate approach for this study, the study did not fit entirely neatly into a phenomenological mode, if such a clearly definable mode exists, but did involve a blurring of the methodology to include an ethnographic element.

Designing the research

The research methodology in qualitative research, as described earlier, takes on more of a matrix formation than a linear one so it may not be so easily controlled by the researcher. Lincoln & Guba (1985 p 210) described how qualitative research needs flexibility of design so that the research can 'unfold, cascade, roll and emerge'. But again, whilst this has come to be a theme for this research, it is also necessary to temper this with the fact that actually carrying out research is a serious activity, one in which the researcher, while engaging in critically thoughtful processes, must also effectively deal with the practicalities of doing research. Marshall & Rossman (1989 p 45) stated that this meant demonstrating the appropriateness and logic of the qualitative methods for the subject being researched.

In order to design the most appropriate method for the area to be studied it was necessary to critically consider what method of data collection would most accurately provide the most useful material about the area under study and one that would remain true to the essence of the experience as lived by the participants. It was obvious that the participation of patients who needed feeding and were currently experiencing being fed was most useful, as opposed to patients asked to consider what it might be like to be fed by another person or attempt to recall a time when they had been fed. Similarly, the participation of nurses currently working with patients who were being fed would prove to be the most useful for this study. Once the participants had been identified it then needed to be considered how best to gain access to their experiences or their reality. This could be achieved by observation, by interview or by combining both methods.

Feeding was an experience that was directly observable and therefore amenable to this method. However, using this method alone would only access some of the experience. It meant that the researcher could obtain data which were interpreted in a different way to the participants and therefore the validity of the data would be questionable. It was necessary to interview participants to access their thoughts and feelings of the experience to gain a greater and more realistic understanding of the experience as lived by the participants.

Many of the research studies in the literature review, such as those carried out by Norberg and her colleagues, used one or a combination of these methods. For the purposes of this study non-participant observation and interviews with nurse and patient participants were selected. However, a major criticism of Norberg's work is her lack of direct involvement with patients. Norberg used patients as a resource or as informants rather than as genuine participants. This may be because much of her work was with patients with severe dementia and it was not possible to obtain rich and meaningful data through interviewing them. The range of observational methods and their consequences were considered through use of the literature (for example, Field & Morse 1985 pp 75–84, Polit & Hungler 1989 pp 206–213). For example, in deciding to undertake non-participant observation both the advantages and disadvantages of this method were considered as well as the advantages and disadvantages of participant observation. The method was also considered in relation to the epistemological foundations of phenomenology for compatibility.

Observational methods

Observation is not always either totally participatory or non-participatory. Field & Morse (1985 p 76) cited the work of Gold (1958) and Pearsall (1965) to describe four types of observational roles: complete participant, participant-as-observer, observer-as-participant and complete observer. Complete participation was considered not to be suitable. Participant-as-observer was not suitable because the researcher had not negotiated to work as part of the nursing team and was only staying in the clinical areas for short periods of time, although that does not mean that this form of observational method was unsuitable for this study. Had a more ethnographic approach been taken then this form of observation may have been more appropriate as it would have enabled the researcher to experience more of the patient and nursing culture. When researchers work in an observer-as-participant role the majority of the time is spent on the observation, compared with a complete observer where the researcher has no direct social interaction with anyone other than what is required for the observations to be carried out. Although a non-participant observational method was used it more closely resembled an observer-as-participant approach than a complete observer. The researcher did establish social interactions with other nurses and patients before, during and after the periods of observation, although only at an informal and superficial level. Given more favourable resources for this research, it may have been possible to carry out the observations using video, as Norberg and colleagues did in several studies. Using a video does not remove the possibilities of researcher interpretation and it may further distance the researcher from the lived experience rather than enhance it, as the researcher is looking at the lived experience through a camera rather than directly at the experience.

The method used in observation also requires comment. Polit & Hungler (1989 p 206) stated that the unit of observation must be decided upon. This means deciding on what is to be observed and the limits to the observation. In this study the unit of observation was fairly broad as it involved observing the interaction between the nurse and patient, how the nurse fed the patient, the social event and processes during the mealtime and activity in the surrounding room or environment during the mealtime. The method had to be reasonably unstructured to enable the researcher to be open to the collection of so much information but at the same time the method of recording had to be organized or structured so that valuable information was not missed, especially where several events or processes were occurring simultaneously.

The main problem with the observation occurred during the first period of observation when the selected method for recording data did not materialize. It was not a case of it not working because as the observation began it felt right to the researcher to record data in a different way. Originally it was planned that the researcher would write down everything that was happening in short note form on a form that had been devised by the researcher. However, as activity began the researcher immediately found that data were divided into two groups based on whether or not they directly involved the patient under observation or whether they were background or indirect patient-related phenomena.

Interviewing methods

Interviewing was a suitable method for this study as open-ended questions and an open-ended question schedule were to be used, although they were formal in that they were prearranged. Antle May (1991 p 189) did not dismiss structured interviews as being unsuitable for qualitative research but did argue that they were best suited to areas of research where the researcher already knew the salient points of the area being explored.

A completely unstructured interview was considered as a possibility. This sort of interview is one where the researcher has no preplanned framework for the interview and simply records whatever the participants talk about. These tend to be more conversations than interviews (Polit & Hungler 1989 p 193). This approach to interviewing is highly compatible with phenomenological methodology, but however appealing it was, it had to be weighed against certain practicalities. One of the disadvantages of using an unstructured approach to interviewing is that it is very time consuming not only in collecting data but also in transcribing and in analysis of the data. Given the time and financial constraints on this study, an unstructured interview approach was not practical.

As the interviews with participants progressed it became obvious that patient and also nurse participants started to talk about similar experiences. For example, all the nurse participants had negative memories of feeding certain patients which could be influencing their feeding experiences. Patient participants tended to talk about what it was like to eat with other patients. As several participants talked about this issue the researcher then used questions that could focus the participants on their experiences without necessarily leading them to provide this information.

In practice, focusing occurred in several stages which did not necessarily follow on from each other. The researcher would ask a question that was fairly open-ended such as '*Do you enjoy feeding patients?*'. Depending on the response and the direction of the response it was sometimes possible to ask a different level question such as '*Can you tell me about any significant experiences of feeding patients you have had [in the past]?*'. It could be that this question was asked at a later stage in the interview if it was not appropriate for it to follow on from the first question. During some interviews it was appropriate to ask more direct questions such as '*Can you tell me about your worst experience of feeding a patient?*'. In order to achieve consistency it was important to remember to ask as many questions as possible of each participant that would produce useful data. It is a learned skill to achieve a balance between flexibility and consistency in interviewing, as described by Antle May (1991 p 193). During any one response given by participants, several areas of interest to the study can emerge. The researcher has to decide which ones to focus on and which ones to leave until later in the interview or which ones not to follow through. Learning to do this is also a skill researchers using qualitative methods need to develop. It is necessary to reflect carefully during and following interviews to understand why topics are and are not pursued by the researcher. It can be easy to become sidetracked by interesting stories patients tell that may not be connected with the research but appeal to the curiosity of the researcher.

Arriving at and using the most appropriate methods for data collection involved a detailed and critical review of the literature on research methodology and techniques for use in the field. It was discovered that while many notable texts provided lengthy information on the academics of qualitative research and their methodologies, they fell short of providing detailed and meaningful assistance about how to use the methods in the field and how to deal with problems and issues that may arise.

Bracketing

This has been described by Swanson-Kauffman & Schonwald (1988 p 98) as part of the ethics of doing phenomenological research. The imperative in phenomenological research is to accurately describe and/or interpret the lived experiences of the participants depending on the exact phenomenological method employed. The degree of accuracy is also an issue of validity which will be discussed in the appropriate section.

Bracketing can be described as a process whereby researchers discounts their own knowledge, values and opinions about the area being researched. This is necessary to enable the participants to fully express the reality of their experiences (Ray 1985 p 88). Swanson-Kauffman & Schonwald (1988 p 89) are more realistic about the process of bracketing as they say bracketing can only be about *reducing* the researcher's assumptions. Bracketing can never occur completely, as the researcher will always be left with some assumptions that impinge in some way on the research process. For this reason the researcher in this study kept a reflective diary that enabled the critical exploration of any assumptions that were held.

Swanson-Kauffman & Schonwald viewed bracketing as a tool to be used by the researcher to meet the ethical demands of accurately portraying the reality of the lived experience as described by the participants. Achieving bracketing is not possible but the researcher, despite knowing this to be the case, must still keep striving towards it. This requires great belief and motivation. As this researcher found, keeping a reflective diary can assist in bringing to the surface assumptions and opinions that may have otherwise interfered with the research. Carrying out a literature review also assists researchers to clarify their assumptions and opinions about the area being researched. But it can also provide further evidence to verify or cast doubt on some assumptions the researcher may already have which again the researcher needs to critically consider in the light of trying to achieve bracketing.

There are several examples of other qualitative researchers discussing this dilemma in the text by Morse (1991). These proved to be informative when considering this issue. It can be argued that researchers carrying out qualitative research need to un-learn certain norms before they can proceed.

Carrying out the fieldwork

Gaining access to the participants was not difficult. This was partly due to the fact that the identified clinical areas for the research were known to the researcher and were ones in which the researcher had already established informal links. It was also made easier because of the positive attitudes from nursing colleagues about nursing research. Senior nurses were very open and positive about the research being carried out in their clinical areas. The researcher knew the clinical environments, some of the staff and had some insight into the cultures of those clinical areas which was an important consideration in a study such as this. The researcher had to be aware to maintain absolute confidentiality about the research.

Throughout the fieldwork the non-participant observation of the nurse participant and the patient participant during a meal was carried out first. The mealtime observed was usually lunch. This was so in three cases but in two cases the meal observed was supper. This means a total of five different nurse and patient participants were observed. Each observation period lasted for approximately 1 hour with the meals lasting for about 45 minutes on average. This meant that the researcher entered the observation area 15 minutes prior to the actual observation beginning. This was a deliberate technique to allow the researcher to familiarize herself with the environment and allow the participants to clarify any points of concern and for other patients and staff to get used to the idea that a researcher was around. When the mealtime had ended the observer ceased formal observations but remained in the environment and chatted with the nurse and/or patient about arranging a mutually convenient time for the interviews.

The interviews with the nurses and patients all took place following the period of non-participant observation, on the same day. In retrospect it probably would have been more useful to have arranged the interviews for another day. This would have enabled the researcher to reflect on the observation more deeply. Every interview began with the researcher making some opening remarks as to the aim of the study. This was taken from Melia (1986) who used a similar technique. In this study the researcher prepared remarks in advance but talked around them to make the remarks seem more conversational.

Interviews were carried out in an informal conversational style using a semistructured approach. This meant that the researcher had questions that would be asked at some point during the interview but that information from the participants also provided the cues for other questions to be asked. In this way valuable information from the participants was accessed that the researcher might not have thought to include. It also meant that each interview was slightly different. Melia (1986) used a similar approach which she termed as 'interviewing with agendas'. She varied the order of the questions according to how the participants responded. Each participant was interviewed once. It is questionable if this is sufficient to yield quality data. Again, given more resources to carry out this study, it would need to be considered if more than one interview with each participant would produce richer data.

Issues of reliability and validity

The research process in qualitative research is different to that of quantitative research and it is not appropriate to apply traditional techniques for measuring reliability and validity to qualitative research. Swanson-Kauffman & Schonwald (1988 p 104) argue that phenomenological research, although rigorous, is not rigid or prescriptive; therefore considerations of reliability and validity can only be that and cannot be regarded as rules. Field & Morse (1985 p 139) defined reliability as a measure of the extent to which random variations may have influenced the stability and consistency of the results. The same authors defined validity as being the extent to which the research findings accurately represented reality. The former definition appears quantitative in nature. Brink (1991 p 165), whilst not defining the two terms, argued that the primary notion in issues of both reliability and validity is that of 'error'. Brink cited the work of Bailey (1978 p 63) who demonstrated where in the qualitative research process error can occur. For example, it can occur in the formulation of the research question and the problem, sampling and data collection error as well as coding and analysis error. Brink discussed types of error and in particular, she considers constant and random error. These two types of validity will now be applied to this study.

Constant error is error that is repeatedly occurring so that true differences between participants are not evident. This is most likely to occur in two ways, either by participants saying what they thought the researcher wanted to hear or by constantly agreeing or disagreeing with questions. The latter is more likely to happen when questionnaires or closed-question interviews are used and was not applicable to this study. The former type of constant error needs to be considered. It is possible that some participants did say some things that they thought the researcher wanted to hear. It is possible to extract several comments in the data from patient participants about how good the nurses were and how they worked really hard. Two patients (Pat and Sam) did openly say they did not want to say anything that would get the nurses into trouble.

It has to be accepted that the validity of the data needs to be considered because participants may not have been telling the complete truth. However, this does not necessarily invalidate the data totally. Not telling the complete truth does not mean participants were lying or deceiving the researcher but it may mean that they did not provide as much data as they could and therefore the picture of their lived experience is not as rich as it otherwise could have been. If this was the case the validity could have been improved by interviewing participants in more depth and for more than one interview.

Sampling

Sampling needs to be considered as an issue of validity. Ten participants were interviewed in this study, not including the two participants used in piloting work. This is not a large number and had time and resources allowed, further participants could have been recruited into the study. The data collection was not saturated. That is, sufficient data were collected for the purposes of this study but it is probable that further data remain to be collected. It is necessary not to confuse sample size in qualitative research with the importance given to it in quantitative research. There was no attempt made, and indeed it would be inappropriate in a phenomenological study, to generalize findings, so achieving a statistically correct sample size and sample type were not major issues.

In qualitative research, sampling is just as critical as in quantitative research but for different reasons. The quality of the sample determines the quality of the data. As Morse (1991 p 127) correctly stated, there are not many guidelines on sampling procedures in qualitative research. Field & Morse (1985 p 95) suggested there are eight different types of sampling methods that can be used in qualitative research while Morse in 1991 (p 127) discussed four methods of sampling as suitable for qualitative research: purposeful, nominated, volunteer and total population samples. Both these guidelines were useful although they did differ in their presentation. The latter guidelines from 1991 were useful to a certain extent as they gave a structure and a name to the sampling procedure for the research. It was possible to say that the sampling method in this research was 'nominated' as senior nurses selected possible nurse participants and then the nurses selected possible patient participants. But it is reasonable to argue that the sampling was by 'volunteer method' as some senior nurses did not directly approach specific nurses but put up information in their clinical areas in the hope that volunteers would emerge. Regardless of the actual procedure used, all participants had to meet the criterion of being involved in feeding at the time of the research.

Some nurses did volunteer themselves or were selected by their senior nurses as being interested but were not used in the study. The main reason for this was that they did not have a patient who required feeding during the period of data collection. The other reason was that the patient they selected was not willing to be interviewed. This happened on one occasion. A patient who had initially given informed consent to participate in the study decided to withdraw. In order to obtain more numbers of participants and seemingly more data, it would have been possible to use observation only with some patients and omit the interviews. On the surface this may have improved the validity of the data but within the context of the epistemological basis of the methodology, it would have reduced the validity of the data. This is because the researcher would not have been exploring the experience of participants to the full and it would have weakened the phenomenological approach to the study.

The social context in which data are collected has a bearing on the reliability and validity of the data (Field & Morse 1985 p 117). The quality of data collected by observational methods in this study could have been influenced by how much was happening in the social environment at the patients' mealtime. At times the researcher had to concentrate on the nurse–patient interaction but at the same time take notice of some other event or interaction occurring in the environment. The previous experience and skills of the researcher are also an influencing factor.

Transcripts of the interviews and observation data were written up as close to the event as possible to minimize the loss of recall by the researcher. Interview transcripts in a draft form were then given to participants as a means of checking the validity of data. Participants were invited to comment on how accurately the researcher had transcribed the interview. With two patient participants it was not possible to give them the transcripts. There were no serious errors identified by the participants in any of the transcripts. Several of the nurse participants commented on how useful they found it to see what they had said written down and that they had taken copies of the transcript so that they could think more about feeding. It is interesting to note that two of the nurse participants said they did not like what they had said in some areas of the interview and they were shocked by seeing their attitudes come through in the transcripts.

Summary

This section has highlighted the methodology selected for this study and some of the issues connected with the choosing of the appropriate methods for data collection. There were some weaknesses in the methods selected for the study and the way in which they were carried out during the fieldwork.

FINDINGS AND DISCUSSION

The majority of the findings have been presented as extracts from participant interviews, using the words of the participants. Reference has been made to material included in the literature review to verify or challenge the findings. The findings were presented in seven sections as was the literature review. This was done simply to provide some organization and structure to this section and it does not suggest or imply any thematic or other significant findings from the data.

In all the extracts from interviews **I** was used to denote the interviewer and **P** to denote the patient or nurse participant. The names of all participants were changed to protect their identities.

Nutrition

The findings on nutrition were perhaps less direct than data in the following sections. This was because the direction of the study was not specifically focused on nutrition and therefore collection of data was incidental. Some of the participants made indirect reference to their nutritional intake.

I   What would you have done if the nurse had not come into the room?

P   I would have left it and made it look as if I didn't want to eat it . . . I do that sometimes if I can't manage.

I   Do the nurses ever have to put food into your mouth for you?

P   With my breakfast I needed help to eat my corn flakes so I cut them out and now I have porridge . . . I've stopped eating toast because I made a mess with it. Meat as well. The meat is difficult to chew and I can't swallow it.

Patient B [Ron]

This patient said he had stopped eating certain foods because he either found them difficult to eat or because he would need them to be fed to him. It may not be a serious nutritional problem that Ron did not eat toast alone but it may be more serious if, as he said, he did not eat meat and his protein requirements were not met from other foods. Ron had been in hospital over a month. There was no evidence that his nutritional intake had been assessed in any one meal or over a period of time or his weight monitored. Patient D [Dave] stated he ate what was essential, one meal a day, and went without food for the rest of the day because he did not like what he was being given to eat. Several participants commented on the quality of certain foods they were given.

P   I enjoyed that fish. Usually, it's meat – and that involves an awful lot of chewing so I don't enjoy it.

Patient A [Pat]

P   If you have trouble eating they think you want to eat steamed fish and mash every other day and I hate the bloody stuff . . . I'd much rather have burger and chips . . . I have one meal a day if I have to and do without the rest of the time until I go home.

[Dave]

Some of the participants commented indirectly on the nutritional intake of other patients on the ward. The patients seemed concerned that some of the other patients could be going without food, either for a part or all of a meal.

P   The lady in the chair who was asleep, she wasn't eating her meal. I wanted her to wake up because she probably won't get another decent meal until tomorrow.

[Pat]

P   As soon as some of the patients stop they take their plates away from them. I don't know if they've finished or not . . . or if you don't eat or you miss a meal you have to wait until the next one. That man falls asleep [points to man] and he doesn't get anything.

Patient C [Sam]

Steamed fish seemed to appear frequently on the menu. Although it is possibly a coincidental observation and despite the comments made by Dave, steamed fish was served for four out of the five meals observed. It seems from both participants' comments and from observation that patients who missed a meal were not provided with a replacement meal or a substitute, at least not during the presence of the researcher. During the observation of all five patients there was at least one other patient that the researcher observed who missed a meal or the majority of a meal. In the interview with nurse C [Julie] the following conversation took place:

I   How would you know if a patient like Sam had not eaten all their meal or how much they had eaten?

P   The catering assistants would tell us.

I   If they forgot to tell you?

P   It wouldn't really matter if it was only for one day.

I   Do you think that's all right?

P   No but the patients aren't going to starve if they don't eat all of a meal or leave something.

That supported the assumption made in the literature review that nurses worked on a meal-to-meal basis and did not take a longitudinal view of their patients' nutritional status. This was further exemplified by the case of Sam. The experience of Sam is interesting and worthy of discussion. He experienced a stroke about 14 months prior to the interview. At that time his doctor prescribed a liquidized diet due to Sam's poor swallowing ability. The nursing documentation showed no evidence of a swallowing assessment by the nurses or the speech therapist and there is no documented evidence of any assessment by a dietician. As time progressed, when he was at home Sam's wife began to reintroduce food presented in ordinary ways and he gradually regained his swallowing ability until he was able, for example, to eat fish and chips when at home. They seem to have carried out this part of his rehabilitation on their own. Sam commented on the fact that he could now eat solid food much better than he could swallow liquids. However, when he went into hospital for respite care 1 week in every 6 weeks, he was still receiving a liquidized diet. Sam said he disliked the diet.

P   It was all mashed up, which I hate them doing . . . some of them mash it up so much it looks like baby food. I never have it at home like that.

I   Why do they do that?

P   Probably they think I might choke – so they are worried about me. I can't use my hand too well and they're probably trying to make it easier for me. The doctor told them I had to have all my food sorted out – but we stopped doing that months ago [at home].

There was no evidence that any reassessment of his diet or his nutritional status was carried out over a period of 1 year. Although he was receiving a liquidized diet in hospital and it can be assumed that the nursing staff believed he was receiving the same at home, his weight was not monitored nor was he assessed to ensure he was receiving a sufficiently varied diet in sufficient quantities. Neither was his swallowing ability reassessed for changes. Despite the arguments by Buergal (1979) and Gaskill & Pearson (1992) in support of the nursing role in nutritional care of patients, the role of the nurse in this patient's nutritional care was very limited. Finally, there was no documented evidence that the nursing staff had considered that it might be possible for Sam to relearn how to eat. This example bears similarities to the case study by Axelsson et al (1986) that was discussed in the literature review.

Glen and colleagues (1993) comment on the inconsistency of treatment in and between disciplines and the lack of communication in the care of patients with swallowing problems in a rehabilitation unit. In Sam's case there was no evidence of any assessment being carried out by a dietician; however, the dietician or therapists may have relied on referral from nursing staff. These authors noted that in their research there were no standard practices for food and fluid consistency based on swallowing deficit in patients. Data from observations in this study would support this. Julie, the nurse participant, said that when she prepared food for Sam she made it into a 'soft diet'. She used a liquidizer but she did say that some nurses only mashed up the food with a fork. However, the main issue in Sam's case was that he was receiving nutrition in totally inappropriate forms whilst in hospital. The fact that he did not feel able to discuss his needs with the nursing staff will be considered in a later section.

Mealtimes

As stated in the literature review, most of the literature considered mealtimes from the nurses' perspective and not that of the patients. Data from interviews with the patient participants did show that patients regarded mealtimes as significant events but that in all cases mealtimes in hospital were different from meals at home and in most cases patients did not appreciate communal or family-style meals with other patients.

I   How would you feel if the nurses thought it would be good for everyone to sit together at the table and eat their meals?

P   . . . I'd like to be on my own. But if you need to be fed and that's where they put you that's where you have to be fed.

I   Would you say meals were a social occasion for you?

P Not really, not so much as at home. I enjoy my meals at home. I chat to the nurses here but it's mainly just eating my food – I like to be on my own.

[Pat]

P . . . I don't like to eat with other people but I need to see them. They must be visible to me so I can see if they're watching me or not. Eating in public just gets me worked up. I have to sit with my back to the wall so I can see all around me and see who is doing what.

I What about eating in this room? [a 4-bedded room]

P Yes even in here it bothers me. I can't explain it, I just get worked up. I know he needs help as well [points to patient] but I still get worked up.

I What about if you were asked to eat in the day room at the table with some of the other patients?

P I wouldn't like that at all.

I No . . . Can you explain why?

P No, not really, I don't know . . . it's just my system.

[Ron]

P I don't like it but we don't have any choice. That's where the nurses take you. I can't get up and walk away, I can't make a fuss. I have to be fed so I sit at the table. That way the nurse can see to us all . . . well it's just embarrassing.

[Ann]

P Huh! Mealtimes, it's like a bloody factory at lunch times. I tend to sit back and watch. I don't want to sit with a bunch of old people I don't know and watch them mess up . . . or me.

[Dave]

Dave was younger than most of the other patients by 30 years and he resented being in their company. He clearly disliked the idea of eating together with people whom he did not know and those who were older than him. Ann, also much younger than the other patients, preferred not to eat her meals in the company of other patients if she was allowed a choice, whilst Ron would seem to become anxious at having to eat in the close company of others and this reaction could affect his psychomotor skills in eating. Sam said he would like to eat in a place other than by his bed but not directly with other people. All five patients said they did not like eating in the dining areas or they did not like eating their meals with other patients. These data suggest that the assumptions made by many healthcare professionals both in research and in clinical practice need to be further questioned and researched (Ott et al 1990, 1991, Pearson 1989 p 130). There needs to be further research that takes into account the patients' views and feelings about family-style meals. Sam said that he would like to eat in a dining area but not with other people. Perhaps the notion of cafeteria meals, where patients can eat in a communal area but can sit at a table on their own or with a few others at most, needs to be further explored.

The nurses' perceptions of mealtimes differed significantly from the patients'. Generally all the nurses in the study thought mealtimes were a social occasion for patients and that patients probably liked to go into the dining room for their meals. Nurse A [Cathy] was the only nurse to consider that patients may not want this and yet she was observed to bring all her patients to the table. Pat specifically asked to be seated across the room from the dining table and facing away from it.

I   Do all the patients generally eat together?

P   Usually, some patients ask not to eat at the table. I suppose they don't like eating with other patients. Perhaps coming into hospital is bad enough without having to eat in front of others.

I   Do you think patients should eat together?

P   In some ways I do. It would help . . . they could all talk together. It would mean the nurses could easily help everyone.

[Cathy]

P   He usually eats by his bed.

I   Does that concern you?

P   Well it doesn't look good. You probably think I haven't tried to get him into the day room for his supper.

I   Is that important – where he eats his supper?

P   I think he should eat in the day room. That's why it's there.

[Julie]

The other three nurses all stated they felt it was important for patients to mix together at mealtimes unless they were not acceptable. The nurses usually decided who was unacceptable according to how bad they were and how much noise and mess they made at the table. The nurses did not take their cue from other patients but usually from each other. It may be that some of the nurses found feeding some uncooperative patients in the presence of others stressful and removed them to a quiet room. As nurse E [Carol] stated:

P   I hate feeding confused patients. They make so much
fuss . . . sometimes I think to myself 'What must other people think

of this?' I find it difficult to be firm with them in case other patients think I'm being cruel. So I tend to put them on their own. I don't find it so difficult then . . . I can just get on with the job.

All the patients felt their mealtimes were too rushed; Dave felt it was like a factory at lunch times and some of the other patient participants felt there was too much going on around them and that it distracted them from eating. Some of the distractions were from nursing and other staff and some distractions were from other patients. Pat was very sensitive to the fact that other patients may need help eating but as the nurse had to stay with her and feed her all her meal, the nurse was not able to run around and help other patients. Several of the patients said they didn't like the way their food was served out, especially when all the courses came together. Observation indicated that plates could be left out of the patients' reach and some parts of the meal appeared poorly presented. For example, in the cases of both Ron and Sam, jelly and ice cream was semiliquid by the time the patients were ready to eat it. Meals were served out by nurses in all the observations and it appeared to be normal practice for these wards, although Julie did not think serving or supervising meals should be a nursing activity.

The direct supervision of the meals was more variable. Nurses tended to go around checking as opposed to staying with patients and therefore the supervision was superficial. This approach, combined with the task approach to be discussed in a later section, meant that the nurses could not have been aware of the food intake and feeding abilities of the patients. This assertion disputes that of Carr & Mitchell (1991) who stated nurses involved in serving meals were more likely to be involved with other mealtime care needed by patients. The researcher's observations do support those of Coates (1985 p 65) who found that nurses gave a higher priority to other activities during the patients' mealtimes. The researcher observed that in all cases either with the patient under observation or other patients in the observation area, meals were interrupted for the administration of medicines or other nurse-orientated activities. In the case of Ann the nurse stopped feeding Ann her main course at lunch time to go with a doctor and arrange an admission to the ward. Cathy, when feeding Pat, had to act assertively to rebuff another nurse who sat down next to them and started talking about the care of another patient.

Nursing skills

Questioning the patient participants about their perception of the nurses' skills in feeding them was a sensitive area. As the researcher had anticipated, patients were very concerned about not getting the nurses into trouble by what they may say and went to lengths to excuse nursing actions on the grounds that the nurses were very busy and had too much work to do. It was possible to begin to get an insight into patients' perceptions in this area but by no means a detailed indepth account. The researcher would suggest that it would take further interviews with patients to obtain more detailed data in this area.

I   Can you ask for assistance if you need it?

P   I haven't had to yet. Things haven't got that bad. I probably would if it got really bad and I wasn't eating at all.

I   Can you ask one of the nurses to help you?

P   Usually the volunteer lady is around so I will ask her. Sometimes you can ask one of the staff . . . some of them.

I   Some of them?

P   It depends on who it is, on their personalities. Some of them I wouldn't ask. All the nurses are nice. I wouldn't say there is anyone that I didn't like. The nurses here are very busy but they do come in and go out . . . I can't really seem to see them they're in and out so quickly, by the time I look up it's too late.

[Ron]

I   Can you tell me what it's like to be fed?

P   It depends on who is doing it and how they do it . . . more on the who really.

[Pat]

P   That nurse [nurse C] the one who helped me tonight, she's different to the others . . . I don't like it when she's here. The others – most of them are very good . . . she does the same as everyone else but it's just the way she tries to get you to do things I suppose.

[Sam]

Clearly the patients were able to differentiate between the nurses and the skills they had. It could be suggested that the patients were sensitive to the personal skills of the nurses and not just their practical skills. As Pat and Sam indicated, it wasn't necessarily what the nurses did but who the nurse was and how she went about it. Pat was able to give step-by-step details of how she liked the nurses to feed her, how and where to position themselves in relation to her, how to put the food into her mouth and what to do with any spillages they made whilst feeding her. Pat said:

P   . . . it helps if they try and understand what I want them to do for me. I remember once asking for a drink of milk and feeling as if I had to drink it all at once. The nurse said you must have been thirsty but I said I wasn't and that I felt I had to drink it all at once and she left it there . . .

The data indicate that patients felt their mealtimes were too rushed and that they were not given sufficient time between courses to eat their food in a relaxed way that would enable them to have a sense of enjoyment from it and perhaps allow them to feel more able to engage in meals as social events. All the patients, when asked '*What could the nurses do to make feeding you a better experience*', responded by saying the nurses could give them more time so they did not feel as if they were being rushed. The observation data indicated that nurses gave cues to patients to increase their pace. For example, the nurse feeding patient A kept moving to the front of her chair and putting a spoon of food up to the patient's mouth before the patient was really ready for the next mouthful. This happened more frequently with Dave and Ann. Two of the nurses were aware that they had a tendency to do this but the other three did not allude to it at all. All the nurses described mealtimes, especially lunches, as being rushed and Cathy described it as 'fraught'.

Several members of the nursing team and non-nursing staff, namely a volunteer tea lady, the domestic and the porter, would go into Ron's room and ask if the patients had finished yet, often while the patients still had food left on their plates. Each person followed in succession, sometimes 2–3 minutes after the last person. In terms of Ron and his eating speed, he would only have managed to chew and swallow one or two small mouthfuls of food before being again asked if he had finished. The data from patients suggest that nurses were not sensitive to the reasons patients left food on their plates other than the fact that they appeared to have finished eating. For nurse B [Kay] it seemed obvious that if patients wanted help they would ask.

I   How would you know if he needed any help?

P   He'd ask obviously!

I   Do you think Ron feels able to ask for any help he needs?

P   Of course, he's not confused at all.

As the comment from Ron earlier indicated, if he could not manage to eat something he made it look as if he didn't want it and left it on his plate. Dave indicated that:

P   . . . they come around and ask if you've finished. I can tolerate that . . . it's when they grab hold of your plate as if it doesn't matter

> if you have or not. That's what pisses me off . . . once they've
> touched it I can't eat anything else . . . it really makes me sick.

Dave was referring to all the ward staff in this extract. Handling the plate unnecessarily caused Dave not to be able to finish his meal.

The literature review considered the work by Deutekom et al (1991) on plate waste-producing situations in wards. It is possible in this study that food was left on plates because of interruptions and specifically the way in which a variety of staff repeatedly asked patients if they had finished their meals. However, this can only be regarded as an unsubstantiated comment by the researcher. It is more realistic to suggest that food was left on plates because patients did not like the food, because they needed some degree of feeding above a level of assistance they were used to or that they were unable for a variety of reasons to ask for help from the nurses.

P Feeding someone isn't that difficult, is it?

Nurse D [Sue]

P Feeding is just one of those jobs you've got to do. It's boring, takes ages and you have little to show for it.

[Carol]

The nurses did not seem to value feeding as a patient-centred activity that required the use of complex nursing skills. None of the nurses in the study could recall ever being shown how to feed patients, either as students or inexperienced nurses new to a particular client group, and none of them could recall reading up about feeding problems, other than how to tube feed a patient. When the interviewer asked the nurses what sort of nursing interventions they could carry out to help patients with feeding problems the five nurses all responded by talking about either nasogastric or gastrostomy tube feeding.

Nurse–patient relationship

There were some indirect data from the interviews and observations that proved useful. For example, during the observation of Pat the one nurse that stayed in the dining room was the nurse feeding Pat. There was also a nursing student who came into the room. He tended to move between several patients to give intermittent assistance with feeding. On two occasions he approached the nurse feeding Pat to ask the names of patients he was feeding. This was on a ward where they had primary nursing. During the observation of Ron, on a ward where primary nursing was also practised, the researcher observed a task-orientated approach to mealtimes and feeding the patients. Eight different nursing and non-nursing staff had an interaction with Ron during his lunch in a total of 17 contacts and within a time span of 35 minutes. Likewise, Ann had five different nursing staff interact with her 15 times over 25 minutes. These findings would support two of the arguments the researcher put forward in the literature review.

Firstly, the care of patients during mealtimes, in particular feeding patients, was organized on a task system regardless of the nursing philosophy or the structural organization of nursing care. The task approach affected all the patients in the study, whether it was Ron and Sam who required intermittent assistance or Pat, Dave and Ann who needed total feeding. Secondly, that having a system of primary nursing, as three of the areas had, did not ensure that patients received individualized care during mealtimes. These assertions call into question the assumptions made by Athlin & Norberg (1987), which were also questioned in the literature review on the basis of the evidence they presented. The findings of this study can also be used to question their arguments and conclusions. This research did not consider the level of continuity with nurses feeding the same patients, as the study by Backstrom et al (1987) did. However, two of the patients, Dave and Ann, did state that they never knew who was coming to help them with their meal.

P ... you don't know who is coming, you just have to wait and see and hope it will be OK. I'm usually OK. I'm not forgotten.

I Will you be helped by the nurse who worked with you that day?

P No ... often it's the auxiliaries who come and see to me at lunch time.

[Ann]

All five nurses said they disliked feeding patients. Three of the nurses had a mental picture of the type of patient they most disliked to feed. In one case it was a patient with severe Parkinson's disease and in the two other cases it was patients with severe strokes. All three of these nurses based this picture on previous bad experiences they had had.

P There was a lady with end-stage Parkinson's. She dribbled everywhere – gallons and gallons. I used to hate it so much. Her food would go in and come out again all with gallons of dribble everywhere. In and out, over and over ... You couldn't just watch it, you had to clean it up. Then she coughed and spluttered a lot. She would spray everything out and it would go all over you.

[Cathy]

P   I hate it, it's a personal dislike of mine . . . actually feeding another person is an awful thing to do. It's time consuming but then people have got to eat.
. . . It all started when I was an auxiliary. I used to feed all the patients. They all had to be fed with pureed food and be given a peeled orange each day. I used to have to peel all these oranges and give them. It's an awful memory. I still can't peel oranges, I have to get someone else to do it.

[Kay]

P   I hate feeding confused patients. They never eat what you give them. It doesn't matter what you give them. It doesn't matter what you try to do, how you try to encourage them, they always win in the end.

[Julie]

For Julie 'winning' meant that patients either made a mess with the food and needed to be washed and changed or '*at least cleaned up*' or it meant that the patients left all the food and refused to eat or be fed. For Julie feeding confused patients was becoming a competition between her and the patients. Two other participants described a similar problem in relation to feeding patients who were confused. This may have similarities to the power struggle discussed in the literature review and to the double-bind situations as described by Norberg et al (1980).

None of the nurses felt that their dislike of feeding affected their relationship with patients. Four of the nurses stated they worked very hard to make sure patients could not tell that they disliked feeding. These four nurses all said that they would not opt out of feeding a patient because they disliked doing it. Yet from observation, patient interviews and reviewing the nursing documentation, it seemed that the care patients received was adversely affected. One nurse referred to patients who needed feeding as 'the feeders'. This implied an impersonal approach to the patients and one that is not conducive to individualized patient care. As it was suggested in the literature review, mealtime care for patients who require feeding does not seem to be individualized. This was certainly the case for all five patients included in this study and was observed to be the case for other patients in the ward areas when observation took place.

I   Do you, then, dislike feeding this patient?

P   Mostly, but then we move him around so no one gets him all the time. I don't mind if it's shared out. I don't like feeding him but there are worse than him. It's just a job that needs to be shared out. If every one mucks in then it doesn't affect your relationship with the patient.

[Julie]

P It's so difficult to do anything right for him. He hates being here, so I tend to do what I have to and get on with other things. I suppose I don't know what he wants so I avoid him, if I'm being honest.

[Sue]

All the nurses said that feeding patients took too long and yet the patients' perception of time for their meals was that they were being rushed and not given enough time. When asked, the nurses all correctly estimated how much time they had spent feeding patients. The mean time spent feeding patients during observation for this study was 37 minutes. Some of the nurses, such as Sue, felt they didn't know how to help the patients and their reaction was to avoid them, which further highlighted their lack of skills and the inadequacy of the nurse–patient relationship.

Patient ability

The ability of patients was not always maximized by nursing staff. This may be a reflection of inadequate nursing skills. The extreme example in this case would be that of Sam. The researcher is not making any claims that this example can be regarded as more than that and is certainly not suggesting that this is in any way typical of nursing practice. Patients provided data which indicated how their abilities were being decreased due to nursing actions or inaction in some cases.

P . . . the soup was nice. It would have been better in a cup with two handles otherwise I spill it.

I Do you have such a cup?

P I brought it in with me – it's the one I use at home. In fact I brought two of them to make sure there was always one clean one to use. I struggle if the top isn't on – you see [demonstrates how he needs to hold the cup]. It's my tremors . . . I'm all right sitting like this but as soon as I start to do anything that's it.

[Ron]

During the period of observation Ron tried to drink from the beaker and spilt soup down his chin and the front of his clothes. He left the rest of the soup untouched. At the end of the meal he refused a drink of tea offered by the same member of staff who gave him the soup but several minutes later accepted one from the volunteer. She used his own drinking cup with the handles on both sides.

P They come past and change the way I hold my fork. I like to hold it a different way since my stroke but they – some of them keep telling me I should try to eat properly. Well I don't care as long as I am eating. My table manners are not my strong point any more [laughs].

[Sam]

The experiences of Ron and Sam support the findings of Sandman & Norberg (1988). These authors found that nurses discouraged patients from feeding themselves when the nurse was assisting them. The actions of the nurse, although not directly discouraging Ron and Sam from feeding themselves, could have made it more difficult for them to do so. It could be argued that the nurses' actions reflected the lack of assessment and patient-centred goals for these patients. In Sam's situation the nurse was trying to make the patient conform either to her norms or absolute norms. This is similar to the issue raised by the researcher about the work of Ott et al (1991) who negatively scored patients for eating peas with their knife.

The data from some of the observations verified the patients' comments. Nurses had a tendency not to see that the right aids and equipment were available at the start of meals. Items like plate guards, non-slip mats, small teaspoons and napkins had to be found after the patients had been given their meals so while nursing staff were locating these items the patients' meals were left in front of them getting cold. Often plate guards were put on the wrong way for the patients to use them or different nurses attending to the same patient would move it around the plate during the same meal.

It became clear from reading and studying the patient interview transcripts that losing the ability to feed oneself and accepting the need to be fed is a complex issue for patients. It is not a straight-forward decision. Patients in this study appeared to go through a process of altering their diet so that they can continue without being fed. Dave stated:

P   I didn't mind when I needed help to get started – other patients do as well. It was when I needed to be fed. That was different. I knew then that I was different, that I needed more help than most others.

All the patients commented that they felt that being fed was excessive work for the nurses. They all acknowledged that they could see that other patients needed help but they all still felt that being fed by another person was demanding too much. Two of the patients, Pat and Ron, felt that the nurses shouldn't have to feed them. These comments could indicate the degree to which self-feeding is considered an essential social skill and one that is fundamental to being socially acceptable to others. Ron commented:

P . . . it's embarrassing being fed. They shouldn't have to do it. It's really the end when that happens.

The researcher would suggest that this comment gave an indication as to the effect having to be fed had on the quality of life for the patient. This is not to generalize and say therefore it must be the same for all patients. However, it is suggested that there is a need for further research that explores the effect of needing to be fed on the quality of life for patients.

As it was stated earlier by the patients, they would often not finish their food and sometimes go without a meal. Ron and Sam would sometimes leave food rather than ask for help if they weren't too hungry. Apart from the nutritional issues involved it may be that the transition between being self-feeding and requiring to be fed is a time of psychosocial crisis for some patients and they may need to move through a process of coming to terms with accepting help, prior to which they tend to reject that help and would rather go hungry. The model of Erikson (1982) as described by Axelsson et al (1986) and Norberg et al (1987b) could be a useful framework for nurses to develop both in practice and for further research into the meaning patients give to needing to be fed. A recent phenomenological case study of the experience of long-term gastrostomy tube feeding produced findings that illustrated the almost opposing attitudes that can occur in coming to terms with long-term tube feeding (Wilson 1993). This again demonstrates that accepting feeding may be a time of crisis for some patients where they consider almost opposing attitudes and values before they are able to come to terms with being fed.

The environment

It is clear from the information presented in the section on mealtimes that the patients in this study experienced numerous interruptions during the course of their meals. It is reasonable to assume that as the patients shared their rooms with others, some of these patients would also perceive the activities of the staff as interruptions. The majority of interruptions observed by the researcher were unconnected to the patients' meals. On most occasions the interruption was for one nurse to talk to the other about an aspect of nursing work unrelated to the patient. Again, it can be suggested that nurses do not see patients' mealtimes as a significant event.

P It's disgraceful what we do. It's really made me think. To us the patients' meals are just something plonked in the middle of the shift to be got over with as soon as possible.

[Kay]

During observation in all the wards the researcher observed and made notes that nurses not involving themselves in supervising or feeding patients tended to stand and talk in the dining areas, albeit for short periods of time. The researcher also observed that there were patients who probably needed some assistance but were not attended to. The normal practice for the wards seemed to be for a selected number of staff to be allocated to the dining room, usually one or two nurses, to attend to all the patients' needs whilst the other nurses got on with other jobs. However, this was only the researcher's observation and it was not verified by the nurses in any way, although during interviews, two of the nurses indicated that they did see patients' mealtimes as a chance to catch up on jobs that needed to be done. Cathy described her environment as being 'fraught' and she added that the nurses were responsible for this. She felt it must affect the patients but she said it was difficult for anything to be done. The noise in this and one other environment was mainly caused by catering and/or domestic staff clearing away plates and cutlery and tipping waste food into bowls. This was done in the dining area whilst other patients were still eating their meals. None of the environments could be said to be quiet and peaceful except for Sam's. In Sam's case it was because he was the only patient not in the day room. He ate his meal by his bed. However, he would have preferred not to have done so.

Summary

The findings from this research have given an appreciation of the experience of feeding for patients and nurses. It has been demonstrated that needing to be fed is a difficult life experience for patients and one that is not easily facilitated by being in hospital. It has also been highlighted that the routine practice of nurses in the study was not as individualized as it could be. Furthermore, the organization of nursing and in some cases the wards did not facilitate patient-centred care. Mealtimes and feeding patients were not accorded a high priority by nurses but this could be because of a lack of knowledge. Nurses had little insight into how patients perceived feeding and into the significance of mealtimes and eating in hospitals, despite the existence of primary and team nursing systems.

The data as recorded by the researcher have been given priority in the findings as essentially the data comprise the findings. All the data are meaningful in this study. Some discussion has taken place, especially to try and link findings with material from the literature review, where this has been appropriate. It was never the intention of the researcher to completely revisit the literature review in light of findings from the study. The researcher has been careful not to spoil the data by too much interpretation, although it is inevitable that some interpretation has occurred. No attempt has been made by the researcher to suggest that any findings from this study are or should be generalizable to other patients or other wards. Nevertheless, this study has attempted to research a particular issue that is of significance to clinical nursing practice and from a perspective that has not been widely documented before. Therefore the study has significance in that sense.

On reflection, it is easy to see how the study could have been carried out differently. In particular, having written up the findings, it is possible to see that if the researcher had asked a different question or phrased a question slightly differently then the data may have produced more results. However, the study was carried out as it has been presented. The main issues that surfaced for the researcher which were not really explored in the study were how being fed can affect the quality of life for patients and the issue of privacy and feeding. With the latter, it gradually occurred to the researcher that patients who needed feeding had little or no privacy when they ate or were being fed, yet feeding someone is a very personal event. For some patients with chewing and swallowing problems it involves invading their bodies and it may involve them spilling food and fluid from their bodies in various forms and yet this is not generally considered to need privacy. Other forms of personal care that involve invading the body are usually done in private. The researcher is not suggesting that all patients who need feeding are fed behind screens but it may be time to question whether patients should have more choice about the degree of privacy when they need to be fed. Having a quiet environment and no interruptions may be all that is necessary for most patients. Mealtimes and feeding need to be considered from the perspective of the patient if nursing practice is to develop more meaningful ways of helping patients who experience difficulties in feeding themselves. This study and dissertation have contributed to an area of nursing knowledge that has not been well researched or documented, but it is recommended that further research of both a qualitative as well as a quantitative nature is required.

REFERENCES

Anderson J M 1991 The phenomenological perspective. In: Morse J M (ed) Qualitative nursing research: a contemporary dialogue. Sage, London

Antle May K 1991 Interview techniques in qualitative research: concerns and challenges. In: Morse J M (ed) Qualitative nursing research: a contemporary dialogue. Sage, London

Athlin E, Norberg A 1987 Caregivers' attitudes to and interpretations of the behaviour of severely demented patients during feeding in a patient assignment care system. International Journal of Nursing Studies 24(2): 145–153

Axelsson K, Norberg A, Asplund K 1984 Eating after a stroke – towards an integrated view. International Journal of Nursing Studies 21(2): 93–99

Axelsson K, Norberg A, Asplund K 1986 Relearning to eat late after a stroke by systematic nursing intervention: a case report. Journal of Advanced Nursing 11: 553–559

Backstrom A, Norberg A, Norberg B 1987 Feeding difficulties in long-stay patients at nursing homes. Caregiver turnover and caregivers' assessments of duration and difficulty of assisted feeding and amount of food received by the patient. International Journal of Nursing Studies 24(1): 69–76

Bailey K D 1978 Methods of social research, 3rd edn. Free Press, New York

Barnard K 1981 Cited in Norberg A, Athlin E 1987 The interaction between the Parkinsonian patient and his caregiver during feeding: a theoretical model. Journal of Advanced Nursing 12: 545–550

Beck C 1981 Dining experiences of the institutionalised aged. Journal of Gerontological Nursing 7(2): 104–107

Brink P M 1991 On issues of reliability and validity. In: Morse J M (ed) Qualitative nursing research: a contemporary dialogue. Sage, London

Buergel N 1979 Monitoring nutritional status in the clinical setting. Nursing Clinics of North America 14(2): 215–227

Carr E K, Mitchell J R A 1991 A comparison of the mealtime care given to patients by nurses using two different meal delivery systems. International Journal of Nursing Studies 28(1): 19–25

Coates V 1985 Are they being served? Royal College of Nursing, London

Cobb A K, Hagemaster J N 1987 Ten criteria for evaluating qualitative research proposals. Journal of Nursing Education 26(4): 138–143

Cumming E, Henry W E 1961 Growing old: the process of disengagement. Basic Books, New York

Davies A D M, Snaith P A 1980 The social behaviour of geriatric patients at mealtimes: an observational and an intervention study. Age and Aging 9(1): 93–99

Deutekom E J, Philipsen H, Ten Hoor F, Huyer Abu-Saad H 1991 Plate waste producing situations on nursing wards. International Journal of Nursing Studies 28(2): 163–174

Erikson E H 1982 The life cycle completed. W W Norton, New York

Field P A, Morse J M 1985 Nursing research: the application of qualitative approaches. Chapman and Hall, London

Gaskill D, Pearson A 1992 The nutritionally vulnerable patient: a pilot study to compare nurses' assessment of intake with actual intake. Journal of Clinical Nursing 1: 101–106

Gendron D 1988 The expressive form of caring. Monograph 2. Perspectives in Caring. University of Toronto, Toronto

Glenn N H, Araya T B, Jones K G, Liljefors J 1993 A therapeutic feeding team in the rehabilitation setting. Holistic Nursing Practice 7(4): 73–81

Judd E 1983 Nursing care of the adult. F A Davies, Philadelphia

Katz S, Akpom C 1976 A measure of primary sociobiological functions. International Journal of Health Services 6(3): 494–507

King N, Goodwin C W, Mason A D 1986 Utilization of nursing staff for assessment of dietary intake. Nutritional Support Services 6(4): 32–35

Kolodny V, Malek A M 1991 Improving feeding skills. Journal of Gerontological Nursing 17(6): 20–24

Lincon L Y, Guba E 1985 Naturalistic inquiry. Sage, London

Lynch-Sauer J 1985 Using a phenomenological research method to study nursing phenomena. In Leininger M M (ed) Qualitative research methods in nursing. W B Saunders, Philadelphia

Marshall C, Rossman G B 1989 Designing qualitative research. Sage, London

Melia K M 1986 'Tell it as it is' – qualitative methodology and nursing research: understanding the student nurse's world. Journal of Advanced Nursing 7: 327–335

Middleton D 1983 Nursing 1. Blackwell, Oxford

Morse J M (ed) 1991 Qualitative nursing research: a contemporary dialogue. Sage, London

Nieswiadomy R M 1987 Foundations of Nursing Research. Appleton and Lange, Norwalk

Norberg A, Athlin E 1987 The interaction between the Parkinsonian patient and his caregiver; a theoretical model. Journal of Advanced Nursing 12: 545–550

Norberg A, Norberg B, Gippert H, Bexhill G 1980 Ethical conflicts in long term care of the aged: nutritional problems and the patient – caregiver relationship. British Medical Journal 280(6): 377–378

Norberg A, Asplund K, Waxman H (1987a) Withdrawing feeding and withholding artifical nutrition from severely demented patients: interviews with caregivers. Western Journal of Nursing Research 9(3): 348–356

Norberg A, Athlin E, Winblad B (1987b) A model for the assessment of eating problems in patients with Parkinson's disease. Journal of Advanced Nursing 12: 473–481

Norberg A, Backstrom A, Athlin E, Norberg B 1988 Food refusal amongst nursing home patients as conceptualized by nurses' aids and enrolled nurses: an interview study. Journal of Advanced Nursing 13: 478–483

Ott F, Reedman T, Backman C 1990 Mealtimes of the institutionalized elderly: a literature review. Canadian Journal of Occupational Therapy 57(5): 162–167

Ott F, Reedman T, Backman C 1991 Mealtimes of the institutionalized elderly: a quality of life issue. Canadian Journal of Occupational Therapy 58(1): 7–16

Pearson A 1989 Therapeutic nursing – transforming models and theories in action. Recent Advances in Nursing 24: 123–151

Perry A G, Potter P A 1990 Clinical nursing skills and techniques, 2nd edn. C V Mosby, St Louis

Polit D F, Hungler B P 1989 Essentials of nursing research, 2nd edn. J B Lippincott, Philadelphia

Pritchard A P, Mallett J (eds) 1992 The Royal Marsden Hospital manual of clinical nursing procedures, 3rd edn. Blackwell, Oxford

Ray M A 1985 A philosophical method to study nursing phenomena. In: Leininger M M (ed) Qualitative research methods in nursing. W B Saunders, Philadelphia

Reeder F 1988 Hermeneutics. In: Sarter B (ed) Paths to knowledge. National League for Nursing, New York

Royle J A, Walsh M (eds) 1992 Watson's medical-surgical nursing and related physiology, 4th edn. Baillière Tindall, London

Sandman O E, Norberg A 1988 Verbal communication and behaviour during meals in five institutionalized patients with Alzheimer-type dementia. Journal of Advanced Nursing 13: 571–578

Sandman O E, Norberg A, Adolfsson R, Eriksson S, Nystrom L 1990 Prevalence and characteristics of persons with dependency on feeding at institutions for the elderly. Scandinavian Journal of Caring Science 4(3): 121–127

Scheflin A E 1975 Cited in Athlin E, Norberg A 1987 Caregivers' attitudes to and interpretations of the behaviour of severely demented patients during feeding in a patient assignment care system. International Journal of Nursing Studies 24(2): 145–153

Swanson J M, Chenitz W C 1982 Why qualitative research in nursing? Nursing Outlook April: 241–245

Swanson-Kauffman K 1986 A combined qualitative methodology for nursing research. Advances in Nursing Science 8(3): 58–69

Swanson-Kauffman K, Schonwald E 1988 Phenomenology. In: Sarter B (ed) Paths to knowledge. National League for Nursing, New York

Tredger J 1982 Feeding the patient – a team effort. Nursing 2: 92–93

Watson R 1990 Feeding patients who are demented. Nursing Standard 4(44): 28–30

Williams J, Copp G 1990 Food presentation and the terminally ill. Nursing Standard 4(51): 29–32

Wilson D 1993 The experience of long-term gastrostomy feeding: a phenomenological case-study. Journal of Clinical Nursing 2(4): 235–242

2

Reviews

SECTION CONTENTS

5. Primary nursing: a feminist perspective   173

6. Spirituality in nursing: towards an unfolding of the mystery   203

7. The most significant 'nothing': a concept analysis of personal space   233

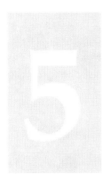

Primary nursing:
a feminist perspective

Rayna McDonald-Birch

Commentary

Disenchantment with structural facets of nursing finds expression in many forms. The well-known problem of sickness rates and feelings of victimization pervade the wards of our hospitals. This discontent is, according to some theorists, about power or its absence. For some feminists, power is centred on gender relations and equity (or indeed, equality) and is achieved through challenges to sex-based power relationships. Those challenges are posed and fought through in real situations in the world of work, the world of the family and in personal relationships.

Primary nursing, as most people are aware, was the thing to do in nursing in the late 1980s and early 1990s. It arose in the United Kingdom for the same reasons that it did in Minnesota, that is as a potential solution to the general dissatisfaction that nurses had with their profession. It promised increased freedom, a sense of individual responsibility and accountability, increased job satisfaction and self esteem, a clearly defined clinical career structure (that was not realized by the promises inherent with clinical regrading) and much more.

Bearing this in mind, it is surprising that nobody really identified a correlation or similarity between primary nursing and some aspects of feminism. Despite all that was written, and it was hardly possible to open a nursing journal during the late 1980s and early 1990s without seeing a paper on the subject, and despite the plethora of research that was performed in the same period, Rayna McDonald-Birch appears to be the first to make comparisons between, for example, the flattened hierarchical structure in primary nursing and some of the basic principles of feminism, the restructured nursing world, identifying that it might be the focus of the power struggle between nurses and between medicine and nursing.

In this undergraduate dissertation, of which parts have been presented at an international conference, but which is printed for the first time here, Rayna takes aspects from contemporary feminist theory, explores the main concepts and values inherent in primary nursing and subsequently is able to draw comparisons between the two. The significance of this is not to be underestimated. This scholarly work identifies that not only might primary nursing be responsible for a variety of changes in patient care delivery and subsequent improvements in clinical care (although the empirical evidence would appear to suggest that the jury is still out on that one), it might also be responsible for the empowerment of women in health care settings and could possibly lead to an increase of awareness by nurses of feminist ideology.

Could it be then, that the 'named nurse' initiative, which replaced primary nursing as the focus of concern in the mid 1990s, may therefore have as much to do with the continuation of patriarchy as it does with improved patient care and communication?

ABSTRACT

The aim of this chapter is to gain insight and understanding into feminism and primary nursing and attempt to identify concepts that are central to them both. It has sought evidence to support the belief that nursing is slowly and possibly covertly beginning to consider feminine values and methods and to question the validity of the current patriarchal culture.

The four main strands of contemporary feminism – liberal feminism, Marxist feminism, radical feminism and socialist feminism – are described and detailed in chronological order. Primary nursing is explained, key elements are identified and discussed. This provides the background information that enables the exploration of the concepts that are central to feminism and primary nursing. Similar trends are identified and their relevance is debated, the position of women in healthcare settings is highlighted and suggestions for strategies for change are given.

In the past, nursing and feminism have never been considered as exponents of one another, yet there is evidence of increased collaboration. Women (including nurses) are beginning to search for a viable escape route from the prison of patriarchy. They are constructing personal and collective philosophies based on the values, beliefs, attitudes and methods of feminism. The conclusion of this review is that primary nursing exhibits many feminist attributes and provides the starting point for nursing to become a profession with a feminist ideology. With the creation of a new reality for nursing there is the potential for praxis. This is described by Wheeler & Chinn (1991) as practice informed by awareness of values, reasons and ethics and for nursing's thinking and ideas to be shaped and changed by experience of these actions.

THE HISTORICAL CONTEXT OF FEMINISM AND PRIMARY NURSING

This is an exploration of feminism and primary nursing. It determines whether they exhibit similar concepts and ideas. Both are relatively immature ideologies and are still developing and seeking a clear direction. Unlike other young disciplines, they do not seek to validate themselves or claim credibility by presenting data in the usual scientific manner. This premise is probably hampering the acceptance of a philosophy such as feminism. At a crude level it is possible to postulate that this is not a reflection of academic rigor but a battle of the sexes.

Feminism is a much used term yet its definition amongst different groups can vary widely. Allan (1993) performed a concept analysis of feminism to clarify its meaning for its use in nursing theory and practice. Following a review of the relevant literature she concluded that the defining attributes of feminism are a concern with gender equality and the promotion of equal rights for men and women; the expression of the above through theory and action and a concern with the individual rather than sexual or biological characteristics or roles. This is a definition of feminism in its broadest terms. It succinctly expresses the fundamental core of all feminism.

Primary nursing was conceived as a result of dissatisfaction with the method of organizing nursing work, which was generally a task allocation method. Primary nursing will be explained in depth in a later section. Briefly, I have taken it to mean that one nurse assesses, plans, implements and evaluates the care of the patient on a 24-hour basis until the patient is transferred or discharged. Primary refers to one nurse having total accountability for a patient's nursing care. When the primary nurse is absent the nursing passes to the associate nurse who maintains continuity of care (Wright 1987).

Nursing and feminism have not been traditional allies yet an exploration of the writing, works and lives of the early nurse leaders reveals a strong feminist perspective. It could be said that Florence Nightingale was an early feminist. In a monograph she wrote entitled *Cassandra* (1852) she protested about women's powerlessness and the waste of 'women's passion, intellect, activity . . .'.

Nightingale recognized that Victorian life stifled any potential for personal growth in the Victorian woman. The roles of wife, mother and hostess were considered the height of social achievement for women of this era. It took Florence Nightingale 9 years of family conflict before she could leave home to start her nurse training (Woodham-Smith 1950). As a result of this conflict Florence Nightingale must have gained much insight into patriarchal culture yet she became the pioneer of an occupation for women that would only increase their bonds and dependence on men. Or is it possible that she envisaged that she was providing women with the potential for empowerment if they wanted it?

Florence Nightingale chose not to align herself with women's suffrage, though she did believe strongly in the cause. It is possible that if she had championed the women's movement at this time, it would have gained more credibility due to her personal prestige and could have influenced nursing practice (Bunting & Campbell 1990). A similar position was adopted by the American Nurses' Association who refused to endorse women's suffrage until 1915. This was explained as being the association's wish to remain neutral. Nursing leaders often chose to reject the women's movement and later feminism and nurture an immature developing nursing profession.

There were several feminist nurses who were active in the women's movement. Such notables include Lavinia Dock, Lillian Wald, Isobel Stuart, Adelaide Nutting and Margaret Sanger. These nurses supported women's right to vote and to control their fertility. They opposed war, worked to help the poor and to educate immigrant women (Mulligan 1993). However, nursing still chose to emulate medicine in the drive for professionalism at the expense of adopting a feminist ideology (Bunting & Campbell 1990).

The women's movement has helped women to become more knowledgeable and assertive as women have learnt to work and relate to each other. Webb (1986) suggested that women want to have more control over their bodies and their health care and to work with healthcare professionals as equal partners. Due to men's attempts to control women and maintain power, women have had knowledge withheld from them and the writing of women's history and activities in all areas have been systematically curtailed. Within personal practice, Webb stressed the importance of sharing knowledge and reclaiming knowledge about health by women (Webb 1986).

Webb links her political analysis of feminism and nursing practice with consciousness by looking at how nurses are prevented from developing a feminist awareness by the doctor–nurse relationship. The subordination and sexism within the relationship and endorsement of it by a patriarchal culture often result in nurses not wanting to embrace a feminist perspective. This leads to nurses being unable to recognize the ways in which women are oppressed in health care because they are women.

AN EXPLORATION OF FEMINISM

Feminism is the only serious and plausible philosophy that provides an alternative to patriarchal thinking and structures. Patriarchy has been assigned many definitions over the years but recently writers in English have defined it as the institutionalization of male dominance over women, rather than a system in which the father holds legal and economic power over the other members of his household, which is the older, more narrow meaning of the term (Kramarae 1993). The fundamentals of feminist thinking are that the two sexes are equal in all significant ways. Feminists also believe that feminine qualities are as valuable and credible as masculine attributes and that these factors require public recognition. Finally feminists believe that there is no dichotomy between public and private life. That is, personal is political and there is no difference in the value structure of either area. The male is in control of both places (French 1985).

Feminism as a philosophical perspective can be divided into many strands. Each division only provides a partial or provisional answer to the questions it addresses. Yet they all equally celebrate womanhood and denounce the oppression, repression and suppression of women in the world today.

Original feminist thought stems from the political theories of liberalism and today most contemporary feminist philosophies have evolved from or in reaction to liberal feminism (Tong 1992). The four main approaches to feminism are liberal, Marxist, radical and socialist (Abbott & Wallace 1990). Other approaches that are less prevalent include psychoanalytic, existentialist, ecofeminist and postmodernist feminism (Humm 1992). A full exploration of these perspectives is beyond the scope of this essay. The four theories considered are not always distinct from one another and overlap frequently.

Liberal feminism

Liberal theory stems from the belief that the individual is allowed by society to be autonomous and to strive for personal fulfilment. It maintains that the rights of the individual are more important than the common good. This means that a system of individual rights is justified because these rights constitute a framework within which we can exercise free choice over our separate 'goods', provided that we do not deprive others of theirs (Tong 1992). Assumptions are based on the realization that there are only limited resources and that the individual (even an altruistic person) has an interest in securing as many of these resources as possible (Tong 1992).

The political challenge is to create a society that allows an individual to strive as he or she wishes to without jeopardizing the welfare of the community. Classic liberalism preserves rights and claims that this provides equal opportunities for all individuals within the market place. Welfare liberals give priority to economic justice rather than civil liberties. They maintain that when the imbalance between persons affects an individual's opportunity the state has to intervene and make adjustments to offset liabilities, so the market place cannot perpetuate these inequalities.

Liberal feminism was originally conceived by Mary Wollstonecraft when she published *A Vindication of the Rights of Women* (1789). In this first major work of feminist scholarship, Wollstonecraft argued that women had to become autonomous decision makers if they were to be economically independent of men. However, she did not propose any strategies for how women were expected to achieve this. She felt that women should be educated on the same basis as men. This would lead women to adopt more masculine traits and to abandon their feminine qualities. She never questioned the value of male traits and constantly advocated reason at the expense of emotion. She stipulated that the distinguishing factor between animals and humans was the ability to rationalize. Her writings ignored that even with a reasonable education women would still face social and legal oppression and could probably only hope at most to win autonomy in domestic and private life. In spite of its limitations and omissions, Mary Wollstonecraft's work laid the foundation stone for feminist theory and the emancipation of women.

The emphasis of liberal feminism lies in the belief that female oppression is a result of the inability of women to succeed in or even enter the public world of academia, politics or economics. This is due to cultural and legal constraints. Liberal feminists want to free women from their oppressive roles that have been used as excuses or justifications for assigning women an inferior position in society. A patriarchal society deems women fit for only certain types of occupations such as nursing, teaching and clerking and that they are incapable of ruling, preaching and investing. A person's biological sex should not have to determine his or her psychological or social gender.

Criticisms levelled at liberal feminism include its lack of consideration for the welfare of the community that is sacrificed for individual freedom (Tong 1992). As their standard they equate 'male being' with human being and male virtues and values with human virtues and values. Liberal feminism has a gender-neutral stance rather than a gender-specific approach (Jaggar & Rothenberg

1984). Elshtain (1981) claimed that liberal feminists overestimate the number of women who want to be like men and abandon their mother role. There is little exploration by liberal feminists into whether gender differences are biologically based and they believe that most differences are culture based (Jaggar & Rothenberg 1984).

Liberal feminism is a very strong movement and it can claim responsibility for most educational and legal reforms that have benefited women. This in turn has led to increased professional and occupational status for women and allowed women to improve the quality of their lives.

To summarize, liberal feminism emerged with the growth of capitalism and proposes equal rights and opportunities for women relative to men and their rights and opportunities. Liberal political theory assumes human beings are essentially rational beings and that 'the fundamental moral values of liberalism are predicated on the assumption that all individuals have an equal potentiality for reason' (Jaggar 1983).

Marxist feminism

The main theme of Marxist feminism is that liberation of women requires the elimination of capitalism. The domestic sphere subordinates women by excluding them from a public productive life (Zaretsky 1974). Marxist feminists recognize that women entering the labour force on its own is not enough for emancipation. Zaretsky (1974) claimed that as long as the family is the major institution in which women participate they will remain oppressed. The solution is to eliminate the family as we know it and to break down the divisions and differences between male and female and work and family. For this to happen women's work has to be considered productive in the same sense that men's work is.

Capitalism oppresses women because much of the work they perform is unpaid. They care for the labour force and raise the next generation of workers. This benefits capitalism and is necessary for its perpetuation (Eisenstein 1984).

A major problem for Marxist feminism is that Marx did not consider the position of women in any of his work. He did not take a neutral stance but chose to ignore or failed to recognize the oppression of women. He adopted a naturalistic approach to the family, implying that women were the main carers in the home (Abbott & Wallace 1990).

Marxist feminists have used the work of Engels (1848) to

develop their theory. Engels argued that the nuclear family was formed in response to a capitalist society. He suggested that the family was a metaphor for the state: the father represents the bourgeois and the mother the proletariat. Men needed to control women in marriage so that men would have legitimate heirs to inherit their property. Women's oppression in the family serves the interests of capitalism.

If women were to gain position in the public sphere, Marxist feminists believe it would be possible for men and women to repair the dichotomy between the private and public worlds capitalism has created (Zaretsky 1974). In this analogy it is capitalism, not men, that is the enemy.

Marxist feminism does not deal with the usual questions associated with feminism such as reproductive and sexual roles. Marxist feminists have focused on the fact that women's work is considered inferior and not real work; how the institution of the family is related to capitalism, and how women are generally given low-paid tedious jobs. Marxist feminists believe that if women's position and function in the workplace can change then the same can happen in the household (Tong 1992). By valuing women's work, society values women and women value themselves.

Radical feminism

Radical feminism is a perspective that is still evolving. The main theme of radical feminism is that women's oppression is the most fundamental form of oppression. This has been interpreted to mean that:

- women were historically the first oppressed group;
- women's oppression is the most widespread and exists in almost every society;
- women's oppression is the deepest in that it is the hardest form of oppression to eradicate;
- women's oppression causes the most suffering to its victims, qualitatively as well as quantitatively, although the suffering may go unrecognized because of the sexist prejudices of the oppressors and the victims;
- women's oppression provides a conceptual model for understanding all other forms of oppression (Jaggar & Rothenberg 1984).

Radical feminism maintains that all women are oppressed by patriarchy, which is a complex system of male domination that pervades all aspects of cultural, domestic and public life. The family is considered to be a major form of oppression for women through sexual slavery and enforced motherhood which stems from male control of women's bodies (Jackson 1993).

Radical feminists do not deny biological differences between men and women but assign different meanings to them. Women's oppression is seen to be based in either the woman's reproductive role or in the male's role as an aggressor, often manifested in the form of rape (Abbott & Wallace 1990). Primarily radical feminism can be seen as a revolutionary movement which fights for the emancipation of women.

One of the first and most important works on radical feminism was Shulameith Firestone's book *The Dialectic of Sex* (1974). Her major claim was that gender differences are so fundamental that they are unrecognized and unchallenged. She argues that not only does women's subordination take place in the traditional areas of employment and education but also in their personal relationships. Firestone believes that gender division is due to biological differences, that women are physically inferior because of their reproductive physiology and because they have to care for a physically helpless infant. This she claims leads to women becoming dependent on men for security. This has been perpetuated by the increasing role of social institutions in childbearing and rearing, the majority of which are male dominated. She advocates that this does not have to be the norm if women were able to exercise choice over when they reproduce and if childrearing was to become a shared occupation with men.

More recently this school of thought has been rejected by contemporary radical feminists who encourage women to recreate a new identity for themselves based on femininity, a celebration of true femaleness. It has been proposed that reproductive biology and associated nurturing psychology are forces that can help to liberate women (Eisenstein 1984). This school of thought is based on the assumption that male biology is to blame rather than female biology. Men are naturally aggressive and can use this to control women (French 1985). This is illustrated throughout history with many examples of men using violence to control women such as acts of Indian suttee, Chinese footbinding, African genital mutilation and American gynaecology (Daly 1978).

A further contemporary radical feminist approach rejects biological explanations. French feminists argue that to give birth is not a natural biological process but that it is a sociohistorical construction (Wittig 1979). Women are forced to believe in practices that are seen to be natural but have led to two distinct biological sexes; this has led to an overgendered society (Delphy

1977). Women are in a separate class because the category 'woman' (and 'man') is a political and economic one; there is a need to eliminate the sex distinction itself. The political challenge is to suppress men as a class. When this disappears, women as a class will as well (Wittig 1979).

One of the major arguments of the radical feminists is that women's culture, knowledge and subjective understanding have all been denied by men. The truths and values in society have all been defined by men. Radical feminists want to change and challenge the way in which knowledge is produced so that women's experiences, values and subjective understandings become a part of this knowledge (Abbott & Wallace 1990). Radical feminists also challenge history and are concerned with discovering 'herstory', the recovery of women's culture and heritage.

Radical feminism does not adequately explain the way in which women are subordinated and exploited by men (Tong 1992). Jaggar (1983) criticized radical feminists for not taking sufficient account of the different forms that patriarchal relationships have taken in different countries and claims that they ignore the differences that exist between the experiences of women from different social classes. Elshtain (1981) feels that the biological explanations employed by radical feminists are reductionist and do not take account of ideology and culture.

Radical feminism has highlighted previous unrecognized abuse of women in the forms of pornography, prostitution, sexual harassment, rape, gynaecology, contraception and abortion (Brownmiller 1975, Daly 1978, Firestone 1974, Millet 1970). Radical feminists have taught women how to celebrate and control their bodies and how to value and use their sexuality and psychology.

Socialist feminism

Socialist feminists have interlaced several threads of other feminist thought to form an ideology referred to as dualism. That is, the analysis recognizes two systems, economics and gender, as being influential. Socialist feminists see the oppression of women as a result of the class system (Deckard 1975). The loss of women's status began with the institution of private property, class divided society, the patriarchal family and state power. The way in which women are controlled in the domestic and public arena has led to their lack of freedom. Emancipation is only possible with the abolition of the sexual division of labour in all spheres of life (Mitchell 1974).

Socialist feminists add a class analysis to their philosophy.

They believe that there are particular problems for working class women and women from ethnic minority groups. They regard the relationship between the personal and public domains as the main factor when defining women. Women are identified by their relationships to a man as a father or husband, rather than on their own merits (Chinn & Wheeler 1985). They view the oppression of women and socioeconomic class oppression as equal factors that mutually reinforce one another.

Women are considered second class citizens in a society founded on patriarchy. According to the analysis of socialist feminism the survival of the state depends upon the exploitation of the working class and of women. It is argued that the owners of the means of production have to change if the experience of the working class and women is to improve (Mitchell 1974).

Socialist feminists consider the economy to include work that does not earn conventional wages such as reproduction, child-rearing and sex, in fact any activity that is not productive (Mitchell 1974). Men have a materialistic interest in women and in order to benefit from this they perpetuate institutional arrangements to ensure their continued domination over women. Socialist feminism relies on the concept of sexual division of labour to explain and investigate relationships between women and their subordination. The ideal is that men and women might disappear as social categories.

Socialist feminism is perhaps the newest of the mainstream feminist theories. This perspective draws on 'the best insights of radical feminism and radical insight' (Jaggar & Rothenberg 1984), believing that human nature is created through biology, society and the physical environment mediated by human labour. It recognizes the relationships between the private sphere of the family and personal life and the public domain of productive work (Chinn & Wheeler 1985). According to this perspective the oppression of women and socioeconomic oppression are equally fundamental and mutually reinforcing.

Conclusions

It is not possible to claim that one theory is correct and others are not but it is important to recognize and appreciate the strengths and weakness of each perspective. Feminism seeks to make visible the experiences of women, to understand their reality. Feminism as a philosophy has uncovered biases, prejudices, distortions and violence as a norm in the social, legal and civil functioning of society. Feminism as an active force aims to liberate women from the many chains that bind them. Feminism as a mission seeks to correct, redefine and create a new equilibrium for men and women to live in.

THE HISTORY OF PRIMARY NURSING

In the past the organization of nursing work has often been a system of task allocation. That is, one nurse performing one task for all patients rather than one nurse fulfilling all the needs of one patient. With this method there is a tendency for the task to be termed basic or technical, leading to the creation of a task hierarchy. Nursing work which was classed as basic or simple, such as washing a patient, would be assigned to junior or un-trained nurses. More complicated tasks such as wound dressing would be allocated to more senior nurses. Several suggestions have been made in order to explain the adoption of this method of organizing work. For example, the practice of adopting rou-tines to produce order has been thought an effective method for reducing work-induced stress and anxiety (Menzies 1960). It has also been felt that adherence to a routine was an effective manner in which to manage work when the workforce was highly mobile, such as when there is a high turnover of staff or bank or agency nurses (Menzies 1960). The gradual realization that both nurses and patients were dissatisfied with this method of delivery of care led to the concept of total patient care.

Primary nursing was first implemented in North America at the University of Minnesota in the late 1960s (Manthey et al 1970). Gradually it began to find its way into the practice and literature of nursing in the United Kingdom (Lee 1979). In international terms the arrival of primary nursing in the UK was rather late. Several countries in Europe as well as Canada, Japan and Australia had already adopted its principles (Wright 1990).

Introducing primary nursing to a ward requires organizational changes, a move away from hierarchical control of practice to in-dependent clinical-based decision making (Binnie 1987). Manthey et al (1970) claimed that the traditional and bureaucratic nurse management has to be broken down for primary nursing to be effective. The alternative, they advocated, is the creation of an environment in which 'individuals feel free to learn, to risk, to make mistakes and to grow'. For such changes to be implemented requires time, vision, leadership and a commitment to change.

Manthey (1980) identified three major problems with the tradi-tional form of the delivery of health care. These were, firstly, that care was fragmented, secondly, that it maintained poor levels of communication and, lastly, that shared responsibility led to a lack of accountability. Primary nursing was a response to these problems, as a new method and philosophy of care that would be delivered in a coordinated, individualistic and comprehensive framework. Complex communication pathways could be broken down into simple, direct pathways to improve effectiveness. Individual responsibility could become clearly allocated.

A DEFINITION OF PRIMARY NURSING

Hegyvary (1982) identified four key concepts on which primary nursing is based:

1. Accountability: the primary nurse is answerable for the nursing care of a patient 24 hours a day throughout the hospital stay.
2. Autonomy: the primary nurse has and acts with authority to make decisions about nursing care of her patients in the mode of self-governance.
3. Coordination: nursing care is continuous around the clock, with smooth uninterrupted flow from shift to shift and with direct communication from caregiver to caregiver.
4. Comprehensive: each caregiver gives all required nursing care to the patient during a specific time period.

The above is a theoretical definition of primary nursing and it is recognized that it would not always be possible for all these criteria to be met (Manthey 1980). However, the concepts outlined above are standards or goals for defining the essence of primary nursing (Hegyvary 1982). As a method of organizing care it empowers patients and nurses so that there is a potential for high-quality care to be delivered within the framework of a partnership (Wright 1990).

THE PHILOSOPHICAL BASE OF PRIMARY NURSING

Manthey, the original exponent of primary nursing, claimed that it is no more than 'a system for delivering nursing care in an organizational facility' (Manthey 1980). Many argue that it has a philosophical base as well as having structural and organizational values (Hegyvary 1982, Manley 1990). Wright (1990) claimed that it is a complete reappraisal of the nurse and the nurse's role. Manley (1990) cites the central philosophy of primary nursing as being the nurse and patient forming a therapeutic relationship.

The quality of the relationship can therefore directly affect the quality of care the patient receives (Tutton 1987).

Those who believe that primary nursing has a philosophical basis often cite humanism as a source. This is not a theory of nursing but rather a philosophical approach which views human beings as a whole with emphasis on the individual's own perspective of their lived experience (McKee 1991). Within this school of thought there is value placed on the subjective experience as it can lead to greater understanding of the individual's personal life and experiences (Hilgard et al 1979).

THE PRIMARY NURSE

Implementation of primary nursing requires a change in the organization of the staffing of a ward. Generally the primary nurse is a registered nurse (Wright 1990), who is responsible and accountable for assessing, planning, delivering and evaluating the nursing care of a group of patients and for making the plans for their discharge (Maguire 1993). The primary nurse may also act as an associate nurse or take responsibility for the management of the ward in the absence of a ward sister (Wright 1990). For the majority of the time the primary nurse acts as the direct caregiver and is responsible for ensuring that all information required for the patient to receive the appropriate care is communicated. The primary nurse has the authority to implement her decisions regarding the nursing care of her patients (Black 1992). Zander (1980) described 12 key elements of the primary nurse's role: accountability, advocacy, assertiveness, authority, autonomy, continuity, commitment, collaboration, contracting, coordination, communication and decentralization.

THE WARD SISTER

The ward sister, although still maintaining the role of team leader, is seen as a source of knowledge and expertise. In primary nursing, the traditional authoritarian role is abandoned in favour of the ward sister becoming an information giver, a coordinator and support giver (Sparrow 1986). Instead of controlling patients' care, the ward sister acts as a facilitator and empowerer for the primary nurses, allowing them freedom to practise and work autonomously (Malby 1988). The ward sister still holds 24-hour accountability for the overall management of the ward and if necessary can take responsibility for a patient caseload in the absence of a primary or associate nurse (Black 1992).

THE ASSOCIATE NURSE

The associate nurse is usually a registered or enrolled nurse, although occasionally student nurses may also take on this role (Black 1992). The role of the associate nurse is to assist the primary nurse in the management of a patient caseload. The associate nurse provides care as prescribed by the primary nurse and generally does not make any fundamental changes to the nursing care plan (Maguire 1993). The relationship between the primary nurse and the associate nurse has been described by Hegyvary (1982) as collegial, with associate nurses retaining responsibility for the care they provide. The importance of the associate nurse role is stressed by many authors, who all feel that there is no place for elitism in the primary nursing team (Maguire 1993, Sparrow 1986, Wood 1990).

KEY CONCEPTS IN PRIMARY NURSING

Accountability

Previously, with traditional methods of organizing nursing care, accountability for the patient was vested in the ward sister, who could then delegate appropriate aspects of care to individual nurses for their span of duty. With primary nursing, one nurse accepts continuous accountability for a patient's nursing needs (Black 1992). Accountability can be defined as being liable to be called to account (*Shorter Oxford Dictionary*, Little et al 1987) or, more specifically, being answerable for one's actions. Bergman (1981) claimed that accountability is composed of three elements: responsibility, ability and authority. This means that the nurse who is being held accountable has to demonstrate the specific knowledge required, has to have been delegated continuous responsibility for the patient and has to have been given the authority to make decisions regarding the patient's care. In the traditional method of nursing these issues are often blurred and this leads to confusion as to which individual is to be held accountable. In primary nursing, authority and overall responsibility are plainly vested in one individual and this consequently delineates clear lines of accountability.

Collegial relationships

As nurses assume new roles within the primary nursing system this has been accompanied by a change in their relationships with patients and colleagues. The essence of these relationships is a mutual feeling of trust and respect (Mead 1990). Primary nursing advocates that the relationship between patient and nurse is one of partnership (Wright 1990). To achieve this primary nurses must be able to treat their patients as equals and learn to negotiate and share control. An example of such a collegial relationship was described by Tutton (1987) who stated how, after spending time talking and listening with Elsie, one of her allocated patients, she gained an insight into her life which 'enabled me to care for her in a partnership and allowed me to make realistic and feasible goals for her daily care and to facilitate discharge plans' (Tutton 1987).

Within primary nursing the role of the ward sister has changed from being directive to being facilitative (McMahon 1990). The role changes to that of a clinical specialist who acts as an advisor to the primary nurse. For primary nursing to be successful primary nurses have to have freedom to be creative when they are planning and prescribing care.

Autonomy

Autonomy can be defined as having the freedom to make discretionary and binding decisions consistent with one's scope of practice. Primary nursing facilitates autonomous practice because it places the authority, responsibility and accountability for a patient's care firmly in the hands of one nurse. In reality, for the primary nurse, professional autonomy means the freedom to construct the patient's care plan independently. Advice can be sought from other professionals but whether it is taken up or not is the choice of the primary nurse (Black 1992). Pursuing autonomous practice not only means greater freedom in the decision-making process but also increases accountability. The decisions the primary nurse makes must be within the realms of their own professional knowledge. For autonomous practice to be a valuable asset to primary nursing, nurses have to develop skills to evaluate the outcomes of their decisions. Johns (1990) claimed that historically, nurses have problems in receiving feedback and in offering it to others. This process is important if nurses are to become aware of their personal capabilities and limitations, an essential requisite if autonomous and accountable practice is going to be successful within the framework of primary nursing.

RESEARCH STUDIES

The Derbyshire study (Bond et al 1991) consisted of a comparative study between a newly opened care of the elderly ward on which primary nursing had been implemented and an established elderly care ward which practised team nursing. The study used Neugarten's Life Satisfaction Survey and the Crichton Royal Behavioural Rating Scale which measures functional behaviour and cognitive functioning. When the two wards were compared the nurses on the primary nursing unit reported experiencing increased job satisfaction and higher levels of stress and at times felt they were not delivering a high enough standard of care. The primary nurses felt that their individual roles were more clearly defined, that there was a greater opportunity for personal and professional development and that they had an increased sense of autonomy and of being valued. With regard to patient outcomes, there was no difference in scores on the Life Satisfaction Scale but patients on the primary nursing unit were more positive about their care. Flexibility of the regime was particularly cited, together with the continual availability and support of a specific staff member. This was a largely descriptive study and relied heavily on direct observation and staff and patient interviews.

Reed (1988) used quality patient scales (Qualpacs) and job satisfaction questionnaires to assess patient care and staff satisfaction on an experimental primary nursing unit. As a control, a unit which employed team nursing was used. The wards were both predominantly elderly care rehabilitative units. It was found that the quality of care was better on the experimental unit. This was shown by a higher Qualpac score on the primary nursing unit. It was also discovered that the nurses on the experimental unit had a different philosophy of care. Their priorities were in favour of the patient and providing individualized care. The nurses on the primary nursing unit showed a higher job satisfaction level. In contrast, it was found that nurses on the ward found their work 'more endless' and uncreative.

The Kingsmead study (Maguire 1993) evaluated the impact of introducing primary nursing on an acute care of the elderly ward. One ward was the experimental ward while a further two acted as control wards. They all had similar attributes, client groups and patient throughput. Many aspects were measured, such as quality of care, nurses' activity, nurses' and patients' views and patient outcomes such as length of stay, mortality, morbidity and discharge patterns.

Quality of care was assessed using Senior Monitor. After a year the ward using primary nursing significantly improved its Senior Monitor score. However, the other two wards had increased their scores as well. It was felt that by implementing a quality assurance programme, all three wards raised their own awareness of quality which resulted in an improvement in quality of care, but the most significant improvement was seen in the primary nursing ward. The study also indicated that after the adoption of primary nursing, nurses had an improved knowledge of patients, better communication and relations with patients and relatives and increased knowledge of and responsibility for specific patients. The nurses working on the primary nursing ward expressed greater job satisfaction than before the changes (Maguire 1993).

Conclusions

From the research literature it is possible to conclude that primary nursing does have the potential to improve patient care. Primary nursing provides a climate for nurses to work in that allows them to exercise their skills and abilities to the utmost. This has resulted in an enhancement in their experience of nursing and improved job satisfaction. Patients have also reported positive feelings towards primary nursing. Outcomes on primary nursing wards, such as mortality rates, length of stay, rehabilitation rates and use of services, were all found to improve (Maguire 1993).

The implementation of primary nursing can prove to be a long and possibly difficult journey. Many barriers may be encountered before successful implementation of primary nursing can be completed. These barriers include underlying resistance to change, lack of motivation, low morale, inappropriate education, changes of roles, unrealistic expectations, medical dominance and lack of preparation (Black 1992). The role of managers is seen as one of facilitating rather than supervising (Ersser & Tutton 1991). The importance of achieving the optimum environment and attitude is recognized as paramount if primary nursing is to flourish and it has been stated that managers should ensure that they are '. . . providing structure without stifling creativity, allowing autonomy without abandoning, teaching without telling and fostering growth without undermining confidence' (Zander 1980). Primary nursing appears to be here to stay and provides a new focus and direction for nurses and an improvement in quality of care for the patient.

CONCEPTS CENTRAL TO FEMINISM AND PRIMARY NURSING

As a result of this exploration of feminism and primary nursing, it could be argued that they share several attributes. These issues will be examined further and an attempt to discover similar trends between these two ideologies will be made.

THE LEGACY OF A PATRIARCHAL CULTURE

Patriarchy has created a value system within our society that has become such a lived reality that few think to question or reject it. The accomplishment of the patriarchal system has been to make men central to society and women marginal (French 1985). In actuality this is a rather hollow achievement as women remain central throughout the world due to their role as mothers. The system of patriarchy has resulted in women being silenced, isolated and marginalized (French 1985).

Nursing is traditionally a female occupation. It is essential to understand oppression if any insight is to be gained into some of the situations and problems that exist in nursing. Roberts (1983) presents an analysis of nurses as an oppressed group. By drawing on feminist and nursing literature and theories of oppression, nurses were shown to exhibit characteristics of oppressed groups. Traits found in nurses are overwhelmingly feminine in their orientation and include compassion, generosity, sensitivity and selflessness. These attributes echo the caring core of nursing. This is mirrored in the insight that feminism affords to the family; the woman's position is one of caring and nurturance, resulting in subservience (Rich 1986). This analogy was carried further by Ashley (1980) who likened the hospital system to that of the patri-archal family; the physician/father dictates to the nurse/mother who cares for the patient/child for little gratitude or remuneration.

Other behaviour exhibited by oppressed groups includes a lack of pride in the group and little inclination to be a part of it. Asso-ciation amongst the members would be considered fruitless as it would merely be a coalition of powerless persons (Roberts 1983). Therefore the oppressed group perpetuates the value system of the dominant group. In a similar manner this is exhibited by nurses in their drive to accrue medically orientated skills and attributes. This is often in an attempt to enhance status, ensure credibility and achieve power. These actions are rarely successful and only serve to perpetuate the patriarchal system (Chinn & Wheeler 1985). Nurses are often unaware that their actions merely serve to oppress them further.

Caring is the fundamental root of nursing's and, to a lesser extent, women's history. Due to the prevalence of the masculine viewpoint, human caring and its inherent femaleness has led to it being 'persistently and consistently devalued publicly, yet privately desired' (Pearson 1991). This had led to caring becoming the invisible commodity of women and more specifically nurses. Nursing has become part of a dominator–dominated system, where women nurses are dominated by male doctors and administrators. The resulting powerlessness and subservience can therefore be directly assigned to gender (Colliere 1986). Caring can have many connotations. It can be viewed as women's work and subsequently invisible or it becomes something to fear as it can threaten power, oppose control and domination and is an evocative reminder of human frailty and factors that are often uncontrollable (Ashley 1980). Colliere (1986) encourages nurses to become more aware of their sociocultural invisibility, so that they can appreciate and recognize their occupational invisibility.

Primary nursing has the potential to provide a platform for change, not only in the delivery of care but in the collective group identity of nurses. A Canadian study (Roberts 1980) discovered that primary nurses were less satisfied with their relationships with their physicians than were team nurses. This was felt to be due to problems that nurses encountered in abandoning their role as doctor's handmaiden. The suggestion was also made that doctors were the main obstacle to this change, in that they were unwilling for their relationship with nurses to change (Roberts 1980). In a British study (Ward 1986), similar problems were encountered in that there were difficulties between primary nurses and their medical colleagues. Yet in this study nurses were wary of changing their approach to care in case it did not receive medical approval (Ward 1986). These differences are perhaps indicative of different cultural factors and that Canadian nurses are more aware of their oppression. It could be argued that British nurses still have to recognize their position as an oppressed group.

AUTONOMOUS DECISION MAKERS

Mary Wollstonecraft, the original liberal feminist, claimed that unless a person can act autonomously he or she is acting as less than a full person. Autonomy is a term much used in feminist (Wollstonecraft 1789) and nursing (Hegyvary 1982) literature but in reality it is perhaps difficult to achieve. Feminists and primary nurses are both striving to become autonomous decision makers (Wollstonecraft 1789, Hegyvary 1982). Autonomy can be defined as the basis of all rights and thereby a legitimate route to power. These two attributes have become gender orientated and nurses in primary nursing networks have to forge a link between the dichotomy of altruism and autonomy if they are to be able to serve others without being subservient (Miller 1991).

Many nurses in the past have recognized that when they embrace a feminist ideology and strive for autonomy and equality they often risk rejecting altruism and caring. Reverby suggested that nurses have to find a language of rights that is communal rather than being based on the individual (1990). This requires nurses to empower themselves and create a political basis for the notion of caring (Colliere 1986).

Several authors claim that within primary nursing the autonomous practitioner remains a hazy notion (Bowers 1987, Salvage 1985). Bowers (1989) claimed that conflict is likely to arise between the primary nurse and ward sister over patient care. The person who is really 'in charge' is the ward sister who holds managerial responsibility and has the potential to exercise this authority. Yet Bowers (1989) also claimed that with primary nursing the ward sister must see a consequent reduction in her authority. These two statements appear to contradict each other. A more constructive way of exploring the shift of autonomy in primary nursing is to consider it as a movement of power from the centre towards a new focus on the patient. This means greater autonomy for all members of the team including the patient (Northcott 1994). This echoes feminist thought as expounded by Wheeler & Chinn (1991), who claim that the feminist alternatives to hierarchy and command are unity and sharing stating that:

The power of unity shares the responsibility for decision making and/ or acting upon those decisions in a lateral network . . . The power of sharing encourages leadership to shift according to talent, interest, ability or skill; emphasizes the passing along of knowledge and skills in order that all may develop individual talent.

EQUAL RIGHTS FOR ALL

Equality has always been a central concept within feminism (Tong 1992). Although women have achieved the vote and acquired full legal and property rights, this did little for women's status in the workforce and did not place women in positions of power. It is only now, nearly 100 years later than these social reforms, that women are beginning to claim a position in society that approaches one of equality, for example as a result of the Sex Discrimination Act. Liberal feminism provides nursing with a political language to argue for rights and equality and it acknowledges that the nurse's right to care should be afforded the same status as the physician's right to cure (MacPherson 1991).

Primary nursing adopts an approach based on equality with colleagues and patients (Wright 1990). Partnership is the key word, whether with patients, nurses or other healthcare professionals. With this approach, primary nurses can begin to work as individual and autonomous practitioners, with control over their own working practices.

Primary nursing has been shown to bring together certain interest groups in nursing. White (1985) has concluded that nurses can be divided into three interest groups. Firstly the generalists, who claim nursing is a practical occupation and that academic qualifications are unnecessary. Secondly the specialists, who receive higher education, seek to control their own work and strive for recognition as professionals. Lastly the nurse managers, who form the managerial hierarchy of nursing and who have absorbed bureaucratic values. White claims that in recent nursing history there has been much conflict between these three groups as each one tries to claim supremacy. Primary nursing could provide a common platform for the generalists and the specialists to unite, the generalists because primary nursing puts the first level nurse in a crucially important position and the specialists because of the autonomy it offers (Bowers 1989). The union of these two nursing groups would provide a powerful base with greater political strength than nurse managers. It would encourage more harmonious occupational relations by reducing elitism and giving all nursing groups an equal voice.

It has been identified that equal status is not necessary for equality to exist. It is necessary, though, for both partners to have an equal need of each other and have something to lose, so that both face equal risks (Black 1992).

OWNERSHIP: CLAIMING CONTROL

Ownership is defined as being the fact or state of being an owner (*Shorter Oxford Dictionary*, Little et al 1987). This is not an attribute immediately associated with women or nursing if we consider ownership as a concept rather than its narrower meaning of the ownership of objects. Radical feminists have repeatedly advocated that women are not in control of, nor have rights of ownership over, their own bodies (Daly 1978). Until recently women have legally been the property of men rather than having personal sovereignty over their bodies (Sampselle 1990). The universal acceptance of violence against women is the outcome of this attitude and exists as wifebeating, rape, prostitution and some cultural practices.

Feminist literature has identified a system-based cause; violence against women is considered to be a natural result of the sexist social order (Chapman & Gates 1978). Violence is used by men to gain power over women. Perhaps the most important issue is not whether a man does or does not use violence but rather that many men feel that they are entitled to express their anger in such a way. A sexist social order has resulted in a prevalent attitude of tacit condoning of violence against women. Another manifestation is the tendency of society to blame the victim, which is then reinforced by the healthcare and legal systems (Sampselle 1990). The most destructive outcome of this is when the victim herself believes she is to blame.

In primary nursing the opportunity exists, through the medium of a therapeutic relationship, for nurses to educate patients regarding ownership of their bodies. This does not only apply to women but also men, as all patients become part of a subservient group and demonstrate loss of power and confidence. The primary nurse's role is often one of enabler or facilitator. For patients to claim personal sovereignty over their bodies nurses have to relinquish or share control. The patient and nurse have to learn to negotiate the care needs to be planned and implemented with the patient and nurse becoming partners with equal power. This can be a delicate role for the nurse to uphold as conflict can arise if the parties disagree about the nature of the problem or the anticipated outcome. Both parties have equal opportunity to influence the outcome (Marks-Maran 1978). Therefore patients must be encouraged to state their perceived understanding of their needs and expectations. Nurses then voices their understanding of the problem and realistic goals and then together with patients they discuss and formulate a plan of action (Roberts 1990).

Swenson (1978) claimed that this is an unrealistic process because the professional will always have greater technical and clinical expertise than the patient. However, control does not have to be based on technical expertise or specialist knowledge. Individuals have to learn to foster an attitude or personal philosophy that values their own emotions and perceptions and that is not overawed by an understandable deficit in their knowledge base. The primary nurse can be an instrumental factor in this process which allows individuals to claim control, choice and personal sovereignty over their own bodies if they so desire. This can prove to be a powerful learning process for the nurse and lead to personal as well as professional development.

KNOWING AND DOING

Contemporary feminism values women's voices, ways of knowing and life experiences as well as expressing concern for human justice and equity. There is the potential within nursing for intellectual growth, activism and empowerment (Ruffing-Rahal 1992). Feminism can help to explain many of nursing's collective experiences as a consequence of patriarchy and the subordinate status of women. Feminism could provide the impetus for the nursing profession to become a global network of individual practitioners that complies with the model of constructivist women who:

... aspire to work that contributes to the empowerment and improvement of the goals of others [they] integrate feeling and care into their work ... address burning issues of the day ... and attempt to humanize their cities (Belenky et al 1986).

Such a model applied to nursing would allow the union of personal thought and action within the framework of a collective force. This allows women to achieve a professional identity congruent with their personal self. Jean Baker-Miller (1986) a psychoanalytic feminist, wrote that the major characteristic of women's (as a whole) identity is 'being in relationship'. This means that the relationships and experiences lived by women cannot be isolated. They form a dynamic network of connections that form the basis of decisions and actions.

Nursing presents many gaps between theory, education, management and practice. Fundamentally these are gaps between what we know and what we do. If nursing can begin to express unity in its knowing and doing, nursing theory will begin to evolve from unique perspectives. This is because new and unfamiliar experiences, practices and paradoxes will be revealed that will require clarification or solution.

Primary nursing provides the starting point for nursing to enter a new era. It keeps the expertise of nursing in direct contact with the patient, possibly eventually leading to a greater affinity between what nurses know and what they do. In primary nursing units where nurses are claiming autonomy and accountability this will have to be accompanied by awareness, appreciation and involvement in research. It is necessary that channels are developed so that researchable ideas can be evolved from practice, followed up, tested and incorporated into practice.

By adopting alternative methods of research based on a feminist epistemology, nurses may find a research process that is accessible and encourages questions to be asked and answers sought. Feminist theory upholds personal lived experience as the basis for analysis. Nurses are constant observers of their patients and this is a potential source of data collection. The methods used may include participant observation, small sampling, indepth interviewing, focus groups, action research and grounded theory approaches. Nursing research in general is moving towards a more qualitative approach and this approach captures the more salient features of men and women in society (MacPherson 1983). This type of data is often not revealed when quantitative methodology is used. It is impossible for nursing to be adequately described by quantitative research, as such research fails to provide meaning for practice and direction for the improvement of patient care (Swanson & Chenitz 1982).

The growth of nursing development units, many of which practise primary nursing and have a specific remit to facilitate research, serves to bring research and practice closer (Closs & Cheater 1994). These units actively encourage innovation and employ increasing numbers of clinical nurse specialists, nurse researchers, lecturer/practitioners, quality assurance and audit nurses, all roles that have the potential to enhance the research process.

ACHIEVING PRAXIS

Praxis is defined by Wheeler & Chinn (1991) as 'values made visible through action'. More simply, this can be expressed as 'I know what I do and I do what I know'. In a similar vein Delmar (1986) argued that there are two elements to feminism: action and consciousness. She suggested that feminism means, at its most basic level, that women suffer discrimination because of their sex, their specific needs are unmet and, to satisfy these needs, radical political, social and economic changes are needed in society.

Historically, feminism has been linked with the women's movement in an attempt to restrict its focus. Popular feminism of the 19th century meant action, not thinking or the articulation of ideas, claims, needs or desires. Feminism became stereotyped as 'doing' and campaigning rather than the more threatening thinking. Now as feminism has evolved it has become a conscious political choice and theory rather than simply action directed towards women's issues.

Nursing is still entrenched in a patriarchal culture, yet there is the beginning of an awareness of how patriarchy is affecting nurses and their work (Chinn & Wheeler 1985). In the 1970s women in general became much more aware of their oppressed position and they adopted masculine traits and values and rejected their traditional feminine attributes (Muff 1982). In nursing this was reflected in the era of 'high tech, low touch' nursing. It was a misguided attempt to achieve autonomy, credibility, status and power by emulating male methods and practices.

Now women are learning not to judge using the male baseline as a standard, as they have learnt that this invariably results in the female being equated with the negative. To reduce or eliminate this standard, society must embrace its own femaleness and use this to create a new standard for judgement and decision making. By looking at the world through a new lens there is a chance that discrimination and oppression may become obsolete.

Professional paternalism still controls and dictates the health care we give and receive. Women perpetuate these values and practices which are considered the norm and therefore not questioned. Nursing is now presenting a challenge to the structure and dynamics of the relationships that exist within the healthcare setting. There is a move towards shared knowledge and power and a flattening of the hierarchy. This manifests as the drive towards primary nursing. Primary nursing has evolved from being a method of organizing nursing work into a philosophy of nursing care. Nursing is beginning to value its inherent feminine values and question the validity of the current patriarchal culture. Primary nursing is providing a forum for nurses to work in a way that allows nursing to become an active therapy in its own right.

Primary nursing units are creating nursing-centred units. This provides the potential for new knowledge to be created inductively. If nurses can begin to study their ways of knowing and the basis of their values they will have the potential to begin framing their 'own' individual or collective definitions of practice. The theory–practice gap will become an anomaly and nursing's actions and philosophies will demonstrate congruity.

All perspectives within feminism can contribute to nursing's understanding of its masculine and medical domination. Liberal feminism provides a basis for equality, autonomy and altruism. Radical feminism, the narrowest theory, provides in-sight into femininity that questions all previous held beliefs and presents unlimited change and opportunity for women and their place in society. Socialist feminism provides insight into women's material circumstances and Marxist feminism offers an explanation into women's productive role.

At the conclusion of this literature review it would appear that feminist methods and processes do present a way forward for nursing. Primary nursing is perhaps only the beginning but serves as a useful starting point. It illustrates that radical change can occur and through innovation nurses and patients can be empowered, the ultimate victory being that, after the implementation of primary nursing, patient care and the experience of the nurse demonstrate improvement (Maguire 1993).

In time, if feminist ideology is adopted and upheld by nurses globally, the method of organizing nursing work will be irrelevant. If nurses demonstrate a feminist philosophy in their work then (as we have seen in primary nursing) the care of the patient will always be paramount. Concepts such as power conflicts, the doctor–nurse game, the unpopular patient and the sick role will be replaced with equality, collaboration, conscience, caring and sharing.

Fagin and Diers (1983) write of nursing as being a metaphor, for mothering, intimacy or sex. If nurses as a profession were to unite as a cohesive whole, then nursing would have the power to create its own metaphors that accurately reflect the true nature of nursing. Nursing has to become visionary if it is to be freed from the doldrums it wallows in. Feminism may prove to be the route to a new reality of nursing that is proud to have care as its focus. In creating its own metaphors, maybe nursing will return to auspicious beginnings and see a role model in Florence Nightingale, a feminist, caring, autonomous, heroic, innovative and visionary nurse.

By achieving praxis nursing can become a practice based on actions that are informed by awareness of values, reasons, ethics and thinking and ideas that are shaped and changed by experience of these actions (Wheeler & Chinn 1991).

Nursing – the turning point

For many years we have heard that nursing is at the crossroads. Nursing never seems to get over being at a crossroads. Indeed, nursing has been at a crossroads many times, but instead of taking a new road, leaders in the profession always choose to continue bearing the burden of continuing to live out the subservient role under the patriarchal system, rather than taking a new road that can lead beyond patriarchy. Nursing is no longer at a crossroads, it is at a turning point. It needs to turn away from being the 'token-torturer' of itself and other women. It needs to turn toward the health awaiting women in a woman-defined, woman-created world that lies beyond patriarchal ideas and institutions.

(Ashley 1980)

REFERENCES

Abbott P, Wallace C 1990 An introduction to sociology feminist frameworks. Routledge, London

Allan H T 1993 Feminism: a concept analysis. Journal of Advanced Nursing 18: 1547–1553

Ashley J A 1980 Power in structured misogyny: implications for the politics of care. Advances in Nursing Science 2: 3–22

Baker-Miller J 1986 Towards a new psychology of women. Penguin, Harmandsworth

Belenkey M F, Clinchy B M V, Goldberger N R, Tarule J M 1986 Women's ways of knowing: the development of self, voice and mind. Basic Books, New York

Bergman T 1981 Accountability: definitions and dimensions. International Nursing Review 28(2): 53–59

Binnie A 1987 Primary nursing structural changes. Nursing Times 83(39): 36–37

Black F 1992 Primary nursing: an introductory guide. King's Fund Centre, London

Bond S, Bond J, Fowler P, Fall M 1991 Evaluating primary nursing part 1. Nursing Times 5(38): 35–39

Bowers L 1987 Who's in charge? Nursing Times 83(22): 36–38

Bowers L 1989 The significance of primary nursing. Journal of Advanced Nursing 14(1): 13–19

Brownmiller S 1975 Against our will: men, women and rape. Secker and Warburg, London

Bunting S, Campbell J C 1990 Feminism and nursing: historical perspectives. Advances in Nursing Science 12(4): 11–24

Chapman J, Gates M 1978 The victimization of women. Sage, California

Chinn P, Wheeler C E 1985 Feminism and nursing. Nursing Outlook 33(2): 74–77

Closs J, Cheater F M 1994 Utilization of nursing research: culture, interest and support. Journal of Advanced Nursing 19: 762–773

Colliere M F 1986 Invisible care and invisible women as health care providers. International Journal of Nursing Studies 23(2): 95–112

Daly M 1978 Gyn/ecology: the metaethics of radical feminism. Beacon Press, Boston

Deckard B 1975 The women's movement: political, socioeconomic and psychological issues. Harper and Row, New York

Delmar R 1986 What is feminism? In: Mitchell J, Oakley A (eds) What is feminism? Blackwell, Oxford

Delphy C 1977 The main enemy. Women's Research and Resource Centre, London

Eisenstein H 1984 Contemporary feminist thought. Unwin, London

Elshtain J B 1981 Public man, private woman. Princeton University Press, Princeton

Engels F 1848/1972 The origin of the family, private property and the state. International Publishers, New York

Ersser S, Tutton E 1991 Primary nursing in perspective. Scutari Press, London

Fagin C, Diers D 1983 Nursing as a metaphor. New England Journal of Medicine 30(9): 116–117

Firestone S 1974 The dialectic of sex: the case for feminist revolution. Morrow, New York

French M 1985 Beyond power on women, men and morals. Abacus, London

Hegyvary S 1982 The change to primary nursing: a cross-cultural view of nursing practice. C V Mosby, St Louis

Hilgard E R, Atkinson R L, Atkinson R C 1979 Introduction to psychology. Harcourt Brace Jovanovich, San Diego

Humm M 1992 Feminism – a reader. Harvester Wheatsheaf

Jackson S 1993 Women and the family. In: Richardson D, Robinson V (eds) Introducing women's studies. Macmillan, London

Jagger A 1983 Feminist politics and human nature. Rowman and Allenfeld, New Jersey

Jaggar A M, Rothenberg P S 1984 Feminist frameworks. McGraw-Hill, New York

Johns C 1990 Autonomy of primary nurses: the need to facilitate and limit autonomy in practice. Journal of Advanced Nursing 15: 886–894

Kramarae C 1993 The condition of patriarchy. In: Kramarae C, Spender D (eds) The knowledge explosion: generations of feminist scholarship. Harvester Wheatsheaf, London

Lee M 1979 Towards better care: primary nursing. Nursing Times 75(33): 133–135

Little W, Fowler H W, Coulson T 1987 The Shorter Oxford Dictionary. Guild, London

MacPherson K I 1991 Looking at caring and nursing through a feminist lens. In: Neil R M, Watts R (eds) Caring and nursing: explorations in feminist perspectives. National League for Nurses, New York

Maguire G with Adair E, Botting D 1993 Primary nursing in elderly care. King's Fund Centre, London

Malby R 1988 All you need is thought. Nursing Times 86(19): 46–48

Manley K 1990 Intensive caring. Nursing Times 86(19): 67–69

Manthey M 1980 The practice of primary nursing. Blackwell, Boston

Manthey M, Ciske K, Robertson P, Harris I 1970 Primary nursing – a return to the concept of 'my nurse' and 'my patient'. Nursing Forum 9(1): 65–83

Marks-Maran D 1978 Patient allocation v task allocation: in relation to the nursing process. Nursing Times 74(10): 413–416

McKee C 1991 Breaking the mould, a humanistic approach to nursing practice. In: McMahon R, Pearson A (eds) Nursing as therapy. Chapman and Hall, London

McMahon R 1990 Collegiality is the key. Nursing Times 86(42): 66–67

Mead D 1990 Research report: collegial relationships among primary and associate nurses. Nursing Times 86(42): 68

Menzies I E P 1960 Nurses under stress: a social system functioning as a defence against anxiety. International Nursing Review 7(6): 9–16

Miller K L 1991 A study of nursing's feminist ideology. In: Neil R M, Watts R (eds) Caring and nursing: explorations in feminist perspectives. National League for Nursing, New York

Millet K 1970 Sexual politics. Virago, London

Mitchell J 1974 Psychoanalysis and feminism. Vintage Books, New York

Muff J 1982 Socialisation, sexism and stereotyping: women's issues in nursing. C V Mosby, St Louis

Mulligan J 1993 Nursing and feminism: caring and curing. In: Kramarae C, Spender D (eds) The knowledge explosion: generations of feminist scholarship. Harvester Wheatsheaf, London

Nightingale F 1852/1980 Cassandra. The Feminist Press, New York

Northcott N 1994 Is the role of the sister/charge nurse being devalued? British Journal of Nursing 3(6): 271–274

Pearson A 1991 Taking up the challenge: the future for therapeutic nursing. In: McMahon R, Pearson A (eds) Nursing as therapy. Chapman and Hall, London

Reed S 1988 A comparison of nurse related behaviour, philosophy of care and job satisfaction in team and primary nursing. Journal of Advanced Nursing 13(3): 383–395

Reverby S 1990 The duty or right to care? Nursing and womanhood in historical perspective. In: Abel E K, Nelson M K (eds) Circles of care: work and identity in women's lives. New York Press, New York

Rich A 1986 Of woman born: motherhood as experience and institution. W W Norton, New York

Roberts L E 1980 Primary nursing: do patients like it? Are nurses satisfied? Canadian Nurse 76(2): 20–30

Roberts S J 1983 Oppressed group behaviour: implications for nursing. Advances in Nursing Science 5: 21–30

Roberts S J 1990 Negotiation as a strategy to empower self care. Holistic Nursing Practice 4(2): 30–36

Ruffing-Rahal M A 1992 Incorporating feminism into the graduate curriculum. Journal of Nursing Education 31(6): 247–252

Salvage J 1985 The politics of nursing. Heinemann, London

Sampselle C M 1990 The influence of feminist philosophy on nursing practice. Image: Journal of Nursing Scholarship 22(4): 243–247

Sparrow S 1986 Primary nursing: organizing care. Nursing Practice 1(3): 142–148

Swanson J M, Chenitz W C 1982 Why qualitative research in nursing? Nursing Outlook 30(4): 241–245

Swenson N 1978 Self care, lay initiatives in health. Social Science and Medicine 12(3): 186–188

Tong R 1992 Feminist thought: a comprehensive introduction. Routledge, London

Tutton E 1987 My very own nurse. Nursing Times 83(38): 27–29

Ward M 1986 Primary nursing in psychiatry. Nursing Process Link Magazine winter: 2–3

Webb C 1986 Feminist practice in women's health care. John Wiley, Chichester

Wheeler C E, Chinn P L 1991 Peace and power: a handbook of feminist processes. National League for Nursing, New York

White R 1985 Political regulators in British nursing. In: White R (ed) Political issues in nursing: past, present and future, vol. 1. John Wiley, Chichester

Wittig M 1979 'One is not born a woman' in Proceedings of the Second Sex Conference. Institute for the Humanities, New York

Wollstonecraft M 1789/1975 A vindication of the rights of women. W W Norton, New York

Wood A 1990 Developing a team. Nursing 4(8): 20–22

Woodham-Smith C 1950 Florence Nightingale 1820–1910. Book Club Associates, London

Wright S 1987 Patient-centred practice. Nursing Times 83(38): 24–29

Wright S 1990 My patient – my nurse. The practice of primary nursing. Scutari, London

Zander K 1980 Primary nursing: development and management. Aspen Systems Co, Aspen

Zaretsky E 1974 Socialism and feminism. Capitalism, the family, and personal life. Socialist Revolution 3(1): 83

Spirituality in nursing: towards an unfolding of the mystery

Louise S. Morgan

Commentary

Religion and religious behaviour is, for the stereotypical British person, a difficult topic and one that is usually excluded from polite conversation – just like politics. Yet, whether we are looking at the Judeo-Christian or other traditions, it is very clear that organized religion has much to say about personhood and about care. Whilst humanists, atheists and agnostics disagree about 'God' or 'spirit', all appear to agree that being a person includes something akin to 'spirituality'.

Louise Morgan recognizes this and reinforces the call for nurses to pay more attention to psychosocial aspects of care in this chapter that explores what is potentially a very difficult, challenging and perhaps controversial topic, that of spirituality and spiritual care in nursing.

As Louise explains in the text, a particular view of spirituality was deliberately taken and then comprehensively explored from a practical, nursing perspective, showing how contemporary nursing literature can be used very effectively. Very clear, pragmatic examples of patients' spiritual needs are given and explored from practical and theoretical perspectives. The latter explores definitions, related terms, research on spirituality, spiritual distress and the potential relationship between spirituality and health.

Finally, Louise explores the role of the nurse in the delivery of spiritual care, outlining nurses' responsibilities and giving some timely advice and guidance on the subject. Paying particular attention to the difficulties of performing a 'spiritual' assessment and the difficulties of planning, implementing and evaluating spiritual care, Louise completed her detailed and well structured exploration of the subject by identifying a number of conclusions, including an identification of the need to recognize that individual spiritual requirements may differ, a call for further research, and the suggestion that spiritual care should be a normal and perhaps multidisciplinary activity.

ABSTRACT

One of the greatest myths pervading nursing is the belief that spiritual care is for ministers of religion to provide and only to those holding religious beliefs. However, spiritual care can be given to anyone and nurses can be in an ideal position to offer it if they have the knowledge and skills and are aware of their own spirituality and spiritual needs. The idea of exploring spirituality was born out of the author's concern following a series of pertinent incidences during clinical placements. This seemed to indicate that there was a lack of understanding about religious, cultural and philosophical practices. One only has to look at the small box labelled 'Religion' on assessment sheets for evidence. A Judeo-Christian position is taken, generally because of the literature available and the questioner's own spirituality. However, all belief systems and ideas have been acknowledged and accounted for throughout the text. The main conclusion is that spirituality is a potential area of need for everyone, deserving effective and appropriate care.

INTRODUCTION

What goes on inside a man? (Chapman 1974).

We are presently in a new era of nursing, where the concept of 'holism' has become the fashionable philosophy of care. For years, people have been familiar with the description of the human being as tripartite, possessing mind, body and spirit. Now, however, nurses are faced with the task of grappling with the spiritual in order to give care that is appropriate and holistic. They now have to think a little harder than the old routine of calling in the chaplain or priest in the last moments of life. With today's society of many different religions, cultures and philosophies, the spiritual care which may benefit one person could be inappropriate, even offensive to another.

In order to begin to understand spiritual care, consider the following cases.

An elderly lady lives in a nursing home. She has lived her life, has many memories and now spends day after day very dependent on the nursing staff for her care. Her son has recently died and she feels that she should have gone first. Her occasional outbursts of 'I wish I was dead' are met with glib responses of 'Now, don't be silly!'. What should we say to her?

A man, dying, requests to see his priest. He is called and the patient is able to make his confessions. He is content and dies peacefully the next day with his family around him.

A lady of Asian origin is allowed to keep her undergarment on underneath a surgical gown during an investigative procedure.

A young mother is readmitted following the discovery of malignant nodes in her spine after a remission period from leukaemia. She turns to Catholicism and seeks to make her peace with God, believing that 'this is now the end'. What makes people turn to religion in times like this, when they have had no such strong belief in the past?

An elderly Jewish lady is unconscious and dying. The relatives' only wish is that her body is not washed during the last offices. Their wish is emphasized in every nursing report and observed when the event occurs.

An elderly gentleman, dying of cancer, spends time talking with the night staff each night. He looks back on his life. He regrets that he never married or even settled down, yet he remains a happy and cheerful person, without complaint. He looks forward to seeing his sisters who are coming over from Ireland to visit him, hoping that they will make it in time. What makes one person accept their disease or impending death with more ease than someone else?

The eventual aim of this review is to provide a greater understanding of what spirituality really is and what it means to nurses, if anything at all. Perhaps then one can recognize the processes that are going on in each of the above mentioned incidents and seek to provide appropriate interventions in future cases.

This review also seeks to dispel some of the myths and uncover some truths about spirituality, using research and anecdotal writings on this subject and applying this knowledge to nursing practice.

This literature review has been written using a wide range of sources and opinions, to prevent a biased argument. The reader is, however, reminded that spirituality remains a very controversial area because there are many opinions but few accepted conclusions.

THE SPIRIT AND SPIRITUALITY

Man is not destroyed by suffering, he is destroyed by suffering without meaning (Morrison 1992).

The concept of spirituality is, like death, a seldom discussed subject. This immaterial, intangible dimension to the human being has left us wondering for centuries or as Burnard (1990) stated, 'Human beings seem to have an inbuilt need to invest what they do with meaning'. Throughout our lives we are faced with questions such as 'Is there a purpose to this life, and if so, where did it come from?', 'Is there a soul or spirit and does it belong to some supreme being?' and 'What will happen to it when we die?'.

To begin at the beginning is to attempt to define what the spirit and spirituality actually are. The problem with this is that, as Smith & Bellemore (1988, cited in Harrison & Burnard 1993) identified, 'There are as many definitions as there are people to define it' or as James (1987, cited in Harrison & Burnard 1993) suggested, words and definitions often fall short of explaining the nature of spirituality, since it is more than mere reality but also a 'field of experience with no sharp boundaries'.

Another question is whether the spirit actually exists, for if it does, then spirituality becomes the manifestation of the spirit in our lives, or as Lane (1987, cited in Harrison & Burnard 1993) put it:

The spiritual dimension is life-giving and integrating. The spirit makes humans more than the material reality in which they are surrounded, as well as what makes humans unique from any other being.

On the other hand, spirituality has also been described as a concept in its own right. Harrison & Burnard (1993) argue that spirituality is more of a conscious or unconscious belief, relating individuals to the world, giving definition and meaning to existence. It can also be argued that spirituality is merely a category under which such intangible human concepts as hope, love, purpose and feelings can be neatly slotted.

Love is a key concept used by Clark (1991) in her description of spirituality. She sees it as a description of the soul, stating that it is '. . . the life force that drives us, controls our intuitions, sense of moral values, philosophy, and thus making us what we are' (p 152). Love then becomes the essence of a person's spirituality, whereby man becomes aware of the unity and interdependence of all being and feels related to creation. In the Bible, it is also written that love '. . . bears all things, believes all things, hopes all things, endures all things' (1 Corinthians 13: 7, NKJV).

Other traits of spirituality have also been identified as faith, forgiveness, peace and hope. Another way to consider spirituality is as a literal manifestation of the spirit, just as physiology is a manifestation of the body and emotions are a manifestation of the mind (Heriot 1992). Therefore, the human being becomes tripartite in nature, possessing body, mind and spirit. This might suggest why patients who are otherwise 'healthy' may be far from experiencing wholeness of life (Thompson 1990). To attempt to prove or disprove the existence of one's spirituality or to 'nail down' what it exactly is or encompasses can be a scientific nightmare. Dickinson (1975) concluded that 'The spiritual is opposed to the biological and mechanical'. The implications of this are that it acknowledges the unenviable task facing those trying to produce research into the area with any degree of scientific credibility.

Over the past two decades, there has been an interest in researching near death experiences (NDEs) as an attempt to examine the possibility of a 'spirit realm'. NDEs are a group of phenomena which have been experienced by people who are close to death. There is no universal definition; however, there are certain common characteristics which are described as:

- Peace and a feeling of well-being
- Separation from the body, often 'looking down on what is happening' and encountering deceased loved ones
- Entering darkness or a tunnel
- Seeing and entering a light.

It is important to consider the explanations which have been suggested for such occurrences. Firstly, that there has been a genuine experience which can affect any person. There is no correlation with age, religion, education, social status, sex or psychiatric history (Cole 1993). Physiological explanations have been offered of what happens to the brain near death and during resuscitation. For example, the brain may turn to the visual cortex and memory for the most stable form of input near death. Also, a feeling of well-being and 'floating' can occur as a result of anoxia (Loader 1990).

Critics of these explanations, such as Cole (1993), point to reports of patients having seen things during an NDE, such as the movement of needles on dials, which they could not possibly have reconstructed from hearing or previous knowledge. Also, there are reports of patients who have seen loved ones whom they did not know had died.

Despite the arguments, the most important factor is the profound long-term effect which these experiences have on the individual (Cole 1993). They often affect the spirituality of the person, resulting in a reduced fear of death, feeling of destiny, preciousness of life, reevaluation of priorities and purposes for life and a more positive attitude toward uncontrollable events. However, for some, the experience serves only to reinforce feelings of helplessness and low self-esteem (Greyson 1992). It is also possible that one's spirituality is a dynamic concept, subject to growth and development just as with our physical aspects. Since we are constantly changing our priorities and perspectives with new experiences, it is possible that our spirituality matures as we age. This involves changes of self and self-perception, relationships, place of self in the world and the world's self view (Heriot 1992).

To illustrate, a child would ask 'Who am I?', whereas an adult would ask 'Why am I?'.

Religion also has had much to do with defining spirituality; however, this has often been due to preconceived ideas. Many people think that the two are synonymous and subsequently 'switch off'. Heriot (1992) attempts to dispel the myth by explaining religion as:

. . . an external formal system of beliefs, whereas spirituality is concerned with a more personal interpretation of life and inner resources of people (p 23).

Religion could also be envisaged as a channel or a way of expressing one's spirituality. Thus, one can be spiritual without being religious. This is good for atheists and agnostics, who will give meaning to their lives through different systems. Having no religion does not remove the need for this (Burnard 1988d). However, for the believer, religion provides a system of security in which they can find meaning in their lives and a hope in an afterlife, so that death is no longer seen as the ultimate end.

In contrast, spirituality has been described by writers with strong atheistic ideas. Hegel's theory of empirical philosophy (cited in Ozinga 1990) suggested that the source of God was people themselves and had a strong emphasis on 'at oneness' between people and the world. Marx's concept of man describes the process of 'self-realization', where the essence of man is in himself, a concept comparable to spirituality (Fromm 1966). Later, Fromm (1968) wrote about hope and faith where hope was described as:

. . . an intrinsic element of the structure of life, of the man's spirit . . . This is closely linked with another element of the structure of life: faith. Faith is not a weak form of belief or knowledge; it is the conviction of the not yet proven, the knowledge of the real possibility, the awareness of pregnancy (p 13).

Faith as described by an atheist author has similarities to a description from the Bible, whereby it is 'being sure of what we hope for, and certain of what we do not see' (*Hebrews 11: 1*, NKJV). To summarize, it can be appreciated that spirituality is a name given to what is found at the very centre of our lives, where we search for meaning, love, actualization, hope, peace and acceptance. It therefore functions at a very personal and individual level. As for a spirit, it could be said that it acts as an animation of one's spirituality, whether it has a literal existence or not.

Whatever the conclusions or answers, there arises the question of the significance of spirituality for nurses. If each person has a spiritual part, then it becomes an important factor which must be considered when nursing the individual holistically.

SPIRITUALITY AND RESEARCH

People are primarily in and of the world, rather than subjects in a world of objects (Heidegger, cited in Reed 1994).

The process of 'nailing down' what the spiritual dimension actually encompasses is a supernatural nightmare. To produce research in this area worthy of any degree of credibility, one is inevitably going to run into problems, as well as the risk of 'treading on too many toes'.

Heriot (1992) concluded that most research into spirituality is qualitative, using phenomenological approaches and storytelling. The method of phenomenology was derived from philosophical roots and operates differently from the traditional, experimental, scientific methods (Jasper 1994). In a study by Jasper (1994) of phenomenology, it was stated that:

. . . The criterion of meaning is central to the research method. The research design needs to access the meaning that the experience has for the participant and this needs to be preserved in identifying the essence of the phenomenon (p 311).

Phenomenology does not seek to reveal causal relationships but rather the nature of phenomena as humanly experienced and is a deliberate move away from quantification and hypothesis testing (Parse et al 1985). Data are usually gathered by means of interviews and interrogatory statements which can be written or oral. It is not surprising, then, that this method is so popular in the research of spirituality and religiosity, where there is little to quantify and many of the definitions are still only ideas or observations. Spirituality is a field of human experience, with no clear boundaries, and it could be suggested that phenomenology would be the method of choice.

Other methods, however, can seek to back present findings, facilitating generalization of results and study replication. An example is the use of analytical scales, such as the Herth Hope Index (1990) and the Death Threat Index (Greyson 1992). Conversely, these frameworks have been criticized for creating difficulty in comparing results (Highfield 1992) and whether such scales can accurately measure such a subjective area (Cumming 1993). Yet in conflict with this is a study where research into grief and religious belief was hampered due to a lack of objective measurements from past research (Austin & Lennings 1993).

Another methodology which has been used in this area is triangulation, whereby a combination of methods serves to validate each other, producing a more 'sound' argument. Metaanalysis has also been undertaken, where studies of past literature and the resulting conclusions may serve as a useful measure to reduce the element of bias in individual studies. Ethnography has also been used, where spiritual issues have been observed in the context of a group; for instance, in terminally ill patients. This serves to produce findings which are more specific and applicable to certain areas. From the research information which was obtained for this literature review, it seems clear that the main intent of research in this area is to gain credibility for theories and hypotheses which would otherwise be deemed 'woolly'. On analysis of the research obtained, there were some interesting points raised appertaining to the limitations of studies. Also, some suggestions were found as to where future research should be directed, in order to reduce flaws and utilize findings appropriately.

Studies of research methodology also highlighted some possible causes of error in the analysis of research. Interpretation is a problem when the researcher approaches the phenomenon with his or her own preconceptions and attitudes, which may influence the way in which the data are analysed (Jasper 1994). Also, 'tacit knowledge' is a danger. This is knowledge gained from an interpretation of personal knowledge which is inarticulate, but affects our interpretation of a situation (Polanyi 1962). This may cause the researcher to try to predict what is behind an ambiguous statement which has varied possible interpretations (Barriball & While 1994).

Social desirability is another problem, where respondents give replies which they perceive as being socially acceptable rather than how they really perceive the issue (Barriball & While 1994, Greyson 1992). This 'response set bias' (Cumming 1993) can be due to a fear of disbelief and judgement and may even be so extreme as a fear of being diagnosed mentally ill, as in studies of near death experiences (Loader 1990).

Prereflective experience can also occur, where the participants have reflected upon the issue before responding, possibly dramatically condensing the story or even excluding painful or confidential parts of the experience (Jasper 1994). If all this is not considered, the valuable nuances of information may remain hidden, which might otherwise have given a much richer insight into the experiences of each subject. Such practices as interrater reliability, team analysis (Jasper 1994), and probing ambiguous remarks (Barriball & While 1994) can be used to minimize these inaccuracies.

In past studies it was noted that, regardless of whether terminology referred to spirituality or religion, 'religiosity' (religious behaviour), or some other Judeo-Christian framework was used as a measuring tool (Heriot 1992). It was posited by Clark et al (1991) that this was due to 'probable sociocultural bias' of a white, middle-class nature. They argued that such frameworks were now inaccurate in an increasingly pluralistic society with more diverse philosophical and religious orientations. The next question appertains to the attitudes and opinions of the researcher. Of the actual studies used for this work, only two out of 16 had any open indication of religious allegiance. This obviously does not account for those with a religious background which would not show as part of a title.

The use of closed questionnaires was criticized by Cumming (1993) and Greyson (1992), for limiting the accuracy of findings, since valuable information may not be brought to light through the limited answers. It has also been identified that there is little or no research into specific problems in spiritual care (Copp & Dunn 1993). For instance, there is little supporting the differences between psychological and spiritual health (Mickley et al 1992), the spiritual health of ill persons (Mickley et al 1992), factors contributing to spiritual health and distress (Highfield 1992) and the assessment of and intervention for spiritual needs (Clark et al 1991). Highfield (1992) commented that broad population samples created difficulty in applying findings to specific areas. However, Barriball & While (1994) found that, despite the varied professional, educational and personal histories of many subject groups, the equivalence of meaning itself helped to standardize results and facilitate comparability. Highfield also identified a 'missing link', in the fact that patients and nurses were often studied alone, with little thought on how they affect each other, so there is a danger that nurses are either missing spiritual problems or identifying ones that aren't there, which may lead to inappropriate spiritual care.

These shortcomings have produced research which is difficult to utilize at ward level. Can findings based on a Judeo-Christian framework be used effectively in the care of a Muslim or an atheist? Also, where does the nurse start when there is no indication in present research of how to identify and utilize strategies in practice (Herth 1990)? 'Spiritual research' also seems to be published only in the more learned journals, those related to oncology and palliative care, and not always in nursing journals. Therefore the accessibility of research is a problem and most nurses make do with anecdotal writings on the subject.

Finally, some of the 'remedies' that have been suggested include random sampling techniques (Heriot 1992), standardized frameworks (Highfield 1992), self-awareness (Burnard 1990) and a multidisciplinary approach to spiritual care (Clark et al 1991). Hopefully, future research will 'fill in the cracks' left by its predecessors in this area to produce findings which are easy to understand and apply to clinical practice, so that the readers no longer despair and become spiritually distressed themselves.

SPIRITUALITY AND HEALTH

Hope deferred makes the heart sick, but when the desire comes it is a tree of life (*Proverbs 13: 12*, NKJV)

As previously, a definition of spiritual health is required before discussing the issues involved. More than one is posited since, if describing one's own spirituality is difficult, how much more then to identify the 'spiritual health' of another individual?

At a White House Conference in 1981, 'Spiritual well-being' was defined as:

The affirmation of life, in relationships with God, Self, Community and the Environment, that nurtures and celebrates wholeness (Byrne 1985, cited in Harrison & Burnard 1993 p 10).

The problem with the above definition is that it is neither very clear nor useful. It is an ideal state in which we 'mere mortals' would become very despondent if we tried to attain it as a short-term goal. Spiritual health is a dynamic process, rather than the arrival at a state of perfection (Morrison 1989). This also confirms the idea of a developing nature of spirituality, as discussed earlier. Spiritual well-being is best described by a list of general characteristics or 'signs on the way' (Morrison 1989). Examples may be a sense of inner peace, compassion for others, reverence for life, gratitude and appreciation of unity and diversity. Indicators of these signs include supportive relationships with other people, realistic goals and orientations toward life events, wholesome self-concepts and ethical conduct (Mickley et al 1992).

Mickley et al (1992), in their study of 175 women with breast cancer, concluded that religiousness may help people create meaning and coherence in the world. However, it is the 'type' of religiousness which is important to note. Intrinsic religiousness is a process of internalizing the creed and following it fully, so that it becomes a master motive in life. Extrinsic religiousness, on the other hand, uses a creed to provide security or social stability, in a utilitarian fashion. It was found that intrinsically religious subjects exhibited a higher level of spiritual well-being than those who were extrinsically religious and that the religious component (that is, the relationship with God) was more important to their spiritual well-being. It was also postulated that intrinsically religious persons of any faith/creed could be more psychologically healthy.

What then for the non-religious or non-believer? One of the greatest myths pervading nursing is the belief that spirituality is only for the religious. Individuals may find meaning and purpose in sociology or psychology; for instance, humanism and humanistic psychology suggest that humans are 'existential', in that they are an agent of 'becoming', constantly changing due to environment, upbringing and culture. Spirituality is seen as the human quest for self-fulfilment (Misiak & Stout-Sexton 1973). From this, Maslow devised his concept of self-actualization and hierarchy of needs, discussed later.

Some people have strong political beliefs (Burnard 1986, 1988d). Some do not have any particular strong beliefs at all, yet their life values and the world as they perceive it are all argued as being valid constructions of their spirituality. Any change has the potential to alter the spiritual health or well-being of the individual from the extent of a minor upset to complete despair. Since we talk of physical health in terms of meeting a set of physiological needs and similarly for psychological health, then it would appear reasonable to suggest that spiritual health is also dependent upon a set of 'needs'. Some of the characteristics have already been described, but how does one achieve these qualities? So far it seems very 'black and white' but spirituality can never be so cut and dried, neither can spiritual health be assumed by a process of ticking off the right criteria.

Maslow (1962, cited in Garrett 1991) described a hierarchy of needs pertaining to each individual. Self-actualization is the attainment of one's full potential and a rich and meaningful life (Coon 1988). This is comparable with spirituality and spiritual needs relate to a group of 'meta-needs' which Maslow suggested were sought by individuals in their striving for self-actualization (Maslow 1970, cited in Coon 1988). These include truth (reality), autonomy, meaningfulness and values, justice and individuality. Other spiritual needs which have been identified include forgiveness, relatedness and belonging, the ability to give and receive love and a sense of awe and wonder about life (Heriot 1992).

Hope has also been identified as a major facet of spiritual health in terms of needs (Mickley et al 1992, Simsen 1988), as well as trust (Simsen 1988). As one would expect, no universal definition of hope exists (Herth 1990), yet there has been increasing interest in this field of research. In a study of the meaning of hope for 30 terminally ill patients (Herth 1990), hope was considered as a coping strategy or in other words:

... an inner power directed towards a new awareness and enrichment of being: rather than rational expectations.

This implies a redirection and reevaluation of values and beliefs, to gain strength from a 'new perspective' on the situation. This study also described seven strategies which such patients adopt to preserve hope and thus satisfy hope as a spiritual need. These are:

1. interpersonal connectedness, meaningful shared relationships with others;
2. lightheartedness, non-verbal communication of joy, delight or playfulness. Humour can also redirect fears and anxieties (Ackerman et al 1993);
3. personal attributes – determination ('iron will', completion of aims), courage (sense of triumph), serenity ('purposeful pausing' allowing hope to surface, inner peace);
4. attainable aims, directing efforts at some purpose;
5. spiritual base, presence of active spiritual beliefs and practices provide meaning which transcends human explanations and fosters hope. Faith in 'God's will' facilitated acceptance (O'Connor et al 1990);
6. uplifting memories, recalling positive moments/times to enrich the present moment;
7. affirmation of worth, to be honoured, accepted and acknowledged (Herth 1990).

The 'unhealthy spirit' is commonly described in literature as spiritual pain or distress. The North American Nursing Diagnosis Association (NANDA) has recognized spiritual distress as one of its approved nursing diagnoses. It is defined as:

Disruption of the life principle that pervades a person's entire being, and that integrates and transcends one's biological and psychosocial nature (Kim et al 1991 p 63).

Their list of signs of spiritual distress (Box 1) has an obvious Judeo-Christian framework; however, the points can be adapted to provide indicators of spiritual distress for persons with a wide range of beliefs and backgrounds.

Box 1   Defining characteristics of spiritual distress

1. Expresses concern with meaning of life and death and/or belief systems.
2. Anger towards God (as defined by the person).
3. Questions meaning of suffering.
4. Verbalizes inner conflict about beliefs.
5. Verbalizes concern about relationship with deity.
6. Questions meaning of own existence.
7. Unable to choose or chooses not to participate in usual religious practices.
8. Seeks spiritual assistance.
9. Questions moral and ethical implications of therapeutic regimen.
10. Displacement of anger toward religious representatives.
11. Description of nightmares or sleep disturbances.
12. Alteration in behaviour or mood evidenced by anger, crying, withdrawal, preoccupation, anxiety, hostility, apathy, etc.
13. Regards illness as punishment.
14. Does not experience that God is forgiving.
15. Unable to accept self.
16. Engages in self-blame.
17. Denies responsibility for problems.
18. Description of somatic complaints.

(Kim et al 1991)

Spiritual distress occurs when the values and beliefs of the individual are disrupted (Rew & Shirejian 1993). This can be to the extent that something shatters the view of life once held and interrupts life with devastating effect (Morrison 1992). This 'something' might include the diagnosis of life-threatening illness, job loss and redundancy, bereavement or marital problems. It has the power to destroy the present views that lie at the centre of our being, to create a very deep level of pain and anguish, which can at worst be shattering (Morrison 1992). Several causes of spiritual distress were identified by Burnard (1986). Firstly there is separation – a lifelong process of 'hellos' and 'goodbyes'. If early experiences of this were painful, then he argues that the process becomes more painful and difficult in later life, causing the individual to question the meaning of it all. One of the 'characteristics' of spiritual distress is a feeling of isolation, abandonment and aloneness (Herth 1990, Rew & Shirejian 1993, Morrison 1992). The patient feels alone in his or her situation, where no-one else has suffered or seems to understand. There may even be a physical and/or emotional loss of significant others. Family and friends play an important role in the individual's search for meaning in the situation and in fostering the hope to deal with it (O'Connor et al 1990).

Facing death is another causative factor (Burnard 1986). The diagnosis of serious or life-threatening illness has a potentially enormous impact on an individual's spiritual health. Their values, beliefs, aims and present-day situation come suddenly into focus and must be reevaluated and defined with the 'shadow' of the diagnosis in mind.

It was also suggested that restrictions of choice may be another contributory factor (Burnard 1986). Coupled with this is a feeling of devaluation and loss of personhood (Herth 1990). Sufferers feels as though they are being treated as 'non-persons' of little value. This generates a feeling of loss of control over the situation and so individuals give way to a feeling of helplessness (Rew & Shirejian 1993) which can also then incorporate a feeling of abandonment and isolation, implying a relatedness amongst characteristics. In severe cases a deterioration into a state of 'learned helplessness' may occur (Seligman 1975, cited in Burnard 1986), whereby the extreme negativity becomes a self-fulfilling prophecy, in that distress deepens because it is deemed inevitable and incurable.

Finally, change and lack of change were identified (Burnard 1986). These both can alter the spiritual stability or security of the individual. Frequent or sudden change, such as a diagnosis of cancer, brings about anxiety, as life no longer seems secure. Conversely, no change implies that aims and ambitions are not being sought and achieved; there is neither progress nor recognition. One may sink into helplessness and despair.

On a more specific level, factors such as uncontrollable pain and discomfort (Herth 1990) have also been identified as contributing to spiritual distress. Consider the despair and helplessness experienced by a patient who cannot eat, sleep or move because of pain. If to live means intense, debilitating physical pain, then that existence may seem entirely meaningless. Also, depression, delirium, fear of loss of bodily functions and mental capacity were suggested as some possible factors which may incite suicidal tendencies in cancer patients (Richards 1994). In the list of the characteristics of spiritual distress as identified by NANDA (Box 1), it is interesting to note that some are factors of other physical and psychological states. Sleep disturbances, for instance, may be indicative of depressive illness or pain. Maybe this is due to a 'holistic' or total response of patients to their illness; that is, a reaction of mind, body and spirit. After the death of his wife, C S Lewis (1966) wrote:

Part of every misery is, so to speak, the misery's shadow or reflection: the fact that you do not merely suffer, but you have to keep on thinking about the fact that you suffer.

So when we speak of health, we must speak of it in terms of a system of interdependent facets, namely mind, body and spirit. A disturbance in one aspect can affect or initiate a reaction in the others. Thus, the role of the nurse must be clearly defined to encompass this realization.

THE ROLE OF THE NURSE IN THE DELIVERY OF SPIRITUAL CARE

Caring is a profound act of hope that contributes to the spiritual well-being of others (White 1986, cited in Clark et al 1991 p 76).

If patients have the potential to become spiritually 'ill' then we had better learn how to care for them. So who is most suitable to give spiritual care? Simsen (1988) identified that if there appears to be any sign of spiritual distress in a client, the nurse's response has historically been to call in the chaplain, thus equating spirituality with religion. She argues that this can no longer be considered an appropriate measure, particularly in such a pluralistic society (Clark et al 1991). Also, it is suggested that the nurse is in an ideal position to provide spiritual care (Canis 1992, Herth 1990, Quesenberry & Rittman 1993). This is due to the amount of time that nurses spend with the patient, as compared to medical staff and other healthcare staff; and the nurse–patient relationship which is established, involving a high level of trust and confidence. It has also been found that nurses, through their character, personal attributes and attitudes, are already acting in the realm of spiritual health and providing spiritual care: they just haven't realized it yet (Forbis 1988, Morrison 1989).

Whether nurses should see themselves as the 'right people for the job' in every instance, however, is another matter. Highfield (1992) found that on an order ranking scale of preferred sources of spiritual assistance, nurses were placed fourth on the list out of seven, by both nurses and patients. Higher ranking choices included family and friends, religious ministers and doctors. Despite the trends found it was emphasized that the patients' choice of spiritual caregiver remained highly individual and personal. This also raises the issue of a multidisciplinary approach to spiritual care, where the patient can be viewed as a whole person, with spiritual needs that can affect the physical and psychological aspects. This way, no problem is 'missed' which might otherwise have been left 'staring us in the face' (Morrison 1990a & b). Also, it allows team members to share experiences, skills and knowledge. The success of this would be in the patient receiving spiritual care and support from the most appropriate person for that individual. A team approach by nurses in providing spiritual care is also indicated, so that spiritual interventions are not left to the nurse who planned and initiated them. This means that such interventions are continued when the nurse is off duty. Examples given in literature are mainly of reading the Bible and praying with patients (Canis 1992, Simsen 1988), although there is obviously more to spiritual care than this, which calls for initiative and a little background reading. As a starting point to outline the role of nurses in spiritual care, the International Council of Nurses Code for Nurses (1973) requires the nurse to respect the spiritual beliefs of the client. The Code of Ethics for Holistic Nurses (American Holistic Nurses' Association 1992) recognizes the need for nurses to become *au fait* with various cultural differences and practices. Finally, the UKCC Code of Professional Conduct (1992, part 7) states that nurses must:

... recognize and respect the uniqueness and dignity of each patient and client, and respond to their need for care, irrespective of their ethnic origin, religious beliefs, personal attributes, the nature of their health problems or any other factor.

Having recognized this need for nurses to take up an active role in spiritual care, the nursing theorist Neuman revised her list of four system variables (physiological, psychological, socio-cultural and developmental), to include 'spiritual' as a fifth. This variable is innate within each individual, but it is acknowledged and developed by choice (Pierce & Hutton 1992). In terms of the Neuman systems model, spirituality is seen as another facet through which energy flows in the client system (patient). When illness, loss, pain or grief occur, energy is lost and the spiritual variable is also affected, evoking signs of spiritual distress (Clark et al 1991). The implication of this for nursing was that the spiritual needs of patients must be considered if the care of patients is ever to become truly holistic or, as Burnard (1988a) put it:

If we are committed to holistic care for patients, to ignore the spiritual aspects of care is surely a gross omission. And, if we do not clarify our own spiritual beliefs or lack of them, how can we help those in our care to clarify theirs?

How does one give spiritual care and incorporate it as part of the patient's planned care? As mentioned above, Burnard (1988a) suggested that we cannot even begin to give spiritual care until we are familiar with our own spirituality; where our own beliefs and value systems lie. If we can more clearly understand ourselves, then we can more accurately discern what is happening to others. This can also serve to lessen the perceived threat from the beliefs of others. However, Burnard (1987) also suggested that we may become so secure in our own beliefs that we become closed-minded and less questioning.

The process of self-awareness was described by Burnard (1990) as:

... the gradual and continuous process of noticing and exploring aspects of the self, whether behavioural, psychological or physical, with the intention of developing personal and interpersonal understanding.

Wyatt (1993) describes the process more specifically, stating that:

Self-awareness involves examining and being sensitive to our emotions, self-concept and personality, and being aware of how these are affected by personal stressors. It also includes awareness of physical limits, potentials, body image, bodily sensations and the effects that social relationships have on others and ourselves.

Burnard (1990), however, warns that self-awareness is not the interpretation of thoughts, feelings and behaviour but rather the practice of noticing them as they are and appear. The aspects which need to be considered in order to develop one's self-awareness are thoughts, feelings, spirituality, sensation, sexuality, physical status, appearance, knowledge, dreams, needs and wants, practice/technical skills, verbal activity, non-verbal activity, self in relation to others, values and undiscovered aspects.

Reflection on certain pertinent issues, the use of reflective diaries, self and peer evaluation are all examples of methods which may prove useful in becoming self-aware. Burnard (1988b) also suggested setting aside a regular time with a friend or trusted colleague to discuss problems, which prevents emotions being 'bottled up'. By doing this, emotions are explored rather than being allowed to get in the way.

In order to implement spiritual care as an essential part of a patient's planned care successfully, it must be relevant to the individual, achievable, understood by nurses and patients and, most importantly, agreed upon and wanted by the patient. Spiritual care can be incorporated into the nursing process.

Assessment

As with all needs, if they are to be met in any way, they must first be recognized or assessed. This is easy to do for someone with a physical need; if I have a headache, my need is recognized as a desire for pain relief, thus the intervention would be to take appropriate analgesia – two paracetamol tablets. This is a crude example, but the point is that physical needs and psychological needs (for example, anxiety) are generally more easily recognizable than spiritual needs. How can one tell if a patient is having trouble 'making sense of it all'?

The problem here is how the nurse can implement some form of 'spiritual assessment', when it should be done and how the correct interventions can be derived from this. There is a widespread feeling among nurses that the box entitled 'Religion' on the front of a patient's Kardex is outdated and inadequate. It is also inaccurate, since many anxious patients would rather state 'Church of England' than express a lack of belief (Burnard 1988d). Also, consider the patient being admitted who is anxious about a diagnosis, work, family, financial circumstances and so on. Would such a person be able to give a detailed explanation of how this has affected the source of meaning and values in life and the impact on any religious or non-religious beliefs held to someone they have just met? It would appear that spiritual assessment should be an ongoing process, as a rapport is established between nurse and patient where there is mutual trust and confidence. Simsen (1988) believed that trust and the process of earning the patient's trust were themselves factors which increased spiritual health. Some questions posited by Charnes & Moore (1992) could be used as part of an initial assessment, to establish a foundation on which to build a more detailed, ongoing assessment. These are:

1. Do you have any particular religious practices that we should know about?
2. In order to care for you, what do we need to know about your:
   • daily routines?
   • dietary preferences?
   • observance of the Sabbath and/or any upcoming holiday?
3. Will your hospitalization affect your daily practices?
4. Is there a minister or other person that you would like consulted or contacted?

Appendix I provides useful points for an ongoing assessment. Nurses also need to keep in mind a holistic approach in assessing the patient's spiritual needs, since spirituality can be expressed in all aspects of life, as mentioned previously. Nurses must also respect the patient's wish to refrain from discussion of certain issues or to object to questioning of their spiritual life altogether (Labun 1988).

Once an initial assessment has been made, Morrison (1990a) suggests that spiritual health concerns should be discussed as part of the handover report, although this raises the issue of confidentiality and trust since a patient's spirituality can be a highly personal subject, yet such information needs to be given to the right people to ensure that any needs are met and care is continued through each shift.

Planning

This requires a good knowledge base on the part of the nurse and the permission and cooperation of the patient. In terms of knowledge, there seems to be a lack of awareness amongst nurses concerning differing beliefs and cultural practices, including the diversity of the Christian faith (Green 1991, 1993). There also seems to be a lack of appreciation of differing levels of belief, since not all followers of a particular religion will observe its practices and rituals to the same extent (Robbins 1991). The level ranges from the very deeply committed to the purely nominal. There is also a need for the nurse to become aware of philosophical and political systems and how various historical thinkers have approached the 'ultimate questions in life' (Burnard 1987). This seems a very tall order for the nurse who envisages hours spent ploughing through religious doctrine and philosophy. However, the patient and family are often one of the best sources of information (Green 1993), as are colleagues, chaplains or friends, for instance, who actually follow a belief system.

Planning involves spending time with the patient, identifying spiritual needs which have been made manifest through observation and assessment. Strategies to meet these needs are then identified and this process requires the involvement of the patient. Such needs may not have even appeared yet; however, there needs to be a contingency plan to deal with anything which may arise during the patient's stay. The patient should feel confident that his nurse is genuinely concerned for him and is available to talk to or that a minister or other desired person will be contacted if the need arises. Thus, planning involves obtaining the information necessary to implement spiritual care and identifying the patient's wishes with regard to his care. There must also be a recognition of the potential stressors and factors which may cause spiritual distress and identifying methods and practices which the patient finds useful in promoting relaxation or refocusing beliefs and values. Such methods may include meditation, listening to music, reading religious doctrine or prayer. It is therefore helpful if the nurse is also aware of some methods which may help the client.

Having made appropriate plans for the spiritual care of the patient, one must now look towards implementing these. However, since spirituality covers such a large area with no sharp boundaries and many different aspects, where does one begin?

Implementation

It has been argued that the main resources necessary for nurses to give spiritual care are a 'listening ear and the ability to give attention' (Morrison 1990a). The art of listening has also been emphasized by many other writers in this field. It is seen as a basic skill which all nurses should be capable of (Burnard 1987, 1988c, Mickley et al 1992). Listening is not, however, as straighforward as it seems. It involves giving attention and demonstrating a genuine concern, rather than appearing nosy or interfering. It also involves observing how the patient tells his story (Burnard 1987). If the patient feels that the nurse accepts him, is genuinely committed without judgement and makes the effort to be approachable and available, this may be enough to initiate a spiritual healing. If the patient has someone that he can tell his problem to, the actual process of talking it through can help him explore the problem. Having undergone a form of reflection on the problem, the patient can then often draw his own conclusions and find his own answers. Thus, the nurse is, albeit perhaps unwittingly, adopting a form of 'catalytic intervention' (Heron 1990). This is one aspect of the 'six Category Intervention Analysis' (Heron 1990), a group of methods adopted in counselling. They are situation dependent to provide the best approach for each client. The first three categories are generally known as authoritative, where the nurse takes on a directive role, appearing 'in charge'; the next three are facilitative, where the nurse is an enabling agent for the patient. It would seem that the latter, facilitative categories would be of most use in helping the spiritually distressed patient.

Touch has been described as a skill which can encourage emotional release (Burnard 1990), especially light touch, such as holding the patient's hand. Heavier touch, such as a hug, can stifle this release and is best used to provide support and comfort after an event. Emotional release can also quite remarkably lift a 'veil' from the problem, enabling the patient to gain a clearer picture of the situation (Burnard 1988b).

In terms of a catalytic response to the need, the use of open questions such as 'How did you feel about that?', as well as echoing (repeating the last few words stated by the patient before pausing, to prompt them in continuing) and picking up on non-verbal cues are indicated in helping the patient make sense of his situation and find his own answers (Heron 1990). The nurse can demonstrate supportiveness by being attentive and available, as mentioned before. There is also a place for appropriate self-disclosure in the management of spiritual distress. Quesenberry & Rittman (1993) describe how the importance of connecting and sharing personal experiences with patients might help them view their distress from another perspective, where they might otherwise have been left feeling alone in their situation.

Reading to the patient has also been indicated (Canis 1992, Forbis 1988). This might be a pertinent passage of religious scripture, poetry or a favourite book. Music can also be soothing and comforting, particularly to those with communication difficulties (Forbis 1988). Prayer can provide a source of comfort and strength (Hegarty 1991, Schneider & Kastenbaum 1993). If this is so, then perhaps nurses have a duty to provide a quiet place where the patient can pray and to be available if the patient asks the nurse to be with them as they pray, if they feel comfortable.

A vital component in the spiritual care of patients is the involvement of family, friends and significant others. They can provide spiritual support (Highfield 1992) or alternatively can be part of the need and may require spiritual care themselves (Taylor & Ferszt 1994). The nurse needs to be aware of the effect of these people on the well-being of the patient and implement strategies to ensure the well-being and involvement of those close to the patient.

In implementing spiritual care, the nurse must also acknow-ledge the role of religious ministers and offer the time, place and privacy to any patient who wishes to speak with the chaplain, priest or religious person of their choice (Copp 1986). Chaplains argue that they would like to become an integral part of the spiritual care of the patient who desires it (Rhodes & Carlisle 1990, Speck 1992) and thus become more recognized as part of the healthcare team. Speck (1992) stated that:

The inclusion of the chaplain into the multidisciplinary team is seen as a recognition of the complex nature of the patient (p 22).

Evaluation

To evaluate, one must look for signs that the patient is regaining spiritual health and is reevaluating his construct and sources of meaning and values.

Colter (1994) describes how a patient who was frustrated by

the diagnosis of terminal cancer, anxious about how his family would cope and in severe pain came to a place of acceptance. After finally managing to control his pain, the nurse sat quietly with the patient for some time. Before getting up to go, the patient said to her:

I finally found out why I have to die . . . My daughter explained it to me . . . According to her, God needs to have the best mechanic in Heaven with Him . . . I guess that's me (p 41).

SPIRITUALITY AND TERMINAL ILLNESS

We all need to leave a mark upon the world as we pass through it, to know that our living has not been in vain (Garrett 1991).

Earlier, it was mentioned that one of the causes of spiritual distress was the diagnosis of life-threatening illness. When a patient receives the 'bad news' their whole life is thrown into turmoil. The job, the family, the house, the ambitions must now come sharply into focus, with the 'shadow' of the illness cast upon each part. If this is true, then terminal illness and the process of dying pose a great threat to the spiritual well-being of these patients.

What the prospect of death means for the individual depends very much upon their spirituality; it is a highly individual experience. What is accepted as a general experience for most dying people is that death is a series of 'losses' (Bolund 1993) which are described as the loss of this present life, 'me', tomorrow, those we love and loss of all we know. In terms of a loss of 'me', this may mean one's sense of identity, autonomy, control (whether actual physical loss of bodily function or control of life events / decisions, etc.), security and of things that are a part of us. Devaluation as a human being was found by Herth (1990) as being a source of hopelessness in terminally ill patients. Loss of control was also found to be a cause of suicidal feelings in cancer patients (Richards 1994). We must therefore be careful, as nurses, to ensure that patients are given as much autonomy and input into their treatment and care as possible, in respect of the patient's wishes. The loss of tomorrow indicates the loss of goals, dreams and ambitions which may never come to fulfilment. Also, it carries the threat of not 'putting things to rights' – where there are unresolved problems or relationships left on bad terms, for instance. This threat to the future can drive people into a stage of 'bargaining' (Kübler-Ross 1970). Bargaining is the third of five stages (denial and isolation, anger, bargaining, depression and acceptance) which a person passes through in the course of terminal illness and dying.

However, it is stressed that people may skip stages, remain 'stuck' at a particular stage or even go through them in a different order. Some may not even appear to be in a stage at all; it is a highly individual process, yet there is a pattern to the general path which people take in the search for meaning and acceptance.

Bargaining is an interesting stage as far as one's spirituality is concerned, since it is at this point when a person's spirituality is most likely to be put into the balance and may be reevaluated or changed. At this stage, the forces of guilt and conscience as the patient reminisces over his life, a longing to see some particular event or just a wish for more time cause the patient to try a new approach. The idea is to gain favour, usually from God or other deity, by undergoing some sacrifice in return. The usual is to promise to go to church more often, give to the poor, donate their body to science in return for more time, less pain, to go to that wedding or even for a cure or miracle. It is important to realize what is behind the 'deal' because it may be due to a fear that God is punishing them for some wrongdoing in their life, for instance, and they may be at risk of a deepening spiritual distress. Bryant (1991) suggests that such people may be comforted and helped by the realization that, according to the Christian faith, God has suffered and continues to suffer and weep with those who suffer.

The trouble with this stage is that it may go unnoticed, since any bargains made are usually in the form of silent determination or secret petitions made to God (Kübler-Ross 1970). Any indications are usually manifested 'between the lines' in conversation or confessed to the chaplain or priest. This again points to the need for a multidisciplinary approach to spiritual care.

Finally, the loss of loved ones can produce much sadness for the patient. This feeling can be held by relatives and friends who realize that they are losing a loved one. Here, the nurse must remember that caring for the spiritual needs of the dying patient involves caring for the family and significant others. As Taylor & Ferszt (1994) put it:

As a nurse, you have a special opportunity to help families cope with a terminal illness. By empowering patients and families to discuss their hopes and fears honestly, you can help promote final healing.

The problem with nursing in this area is that nurses have often been guilty of avoidance behaviour with patients who have a poor prognosis and suffer much anxiety about death (Webber 1993). In a study of 167 nurses involved with the care of the dying (Copp & Dunn 1993), they were asked to identify the five most common problems encountered and the five most difficult to manage. Nine main categories were elicited: physical, work related, death related, emotional, nurse related, communication, family related, losses/changes and spiritual problems. Of these categories, spiritual problems amounted to only 0.1% of the frequent problems perceived by nurses and 0.9% of problems perceived as difficult. This implies that either spiritual problems are only rarely encountered and thus given little priority by nurses or it could be due to a lack of awareness in identifying and recognizing spiritual problems. Copp & Dunn (1993) argue that a reason for this might be the lack of clear guidelines on how to handle spiritual problems.

It has also been argued that an increasingly science-conscious culture has created an image of 'scientific objectivity', where health professionals are taught not to become involved and patients and families expect an 'uninvolved, professional demeanour' (Hampe 1975). More recent research and philosophy seem to be working to remove this myth, but one wonders if such a 'scientific objectivity' is also to blame for a society which seems ill prepared to face death. In a 2-year study of 1000 Italians with a wide range of age, social status, geographical location and religiosity, it was found that death and dying are no longer seen as a natural event in life so that most people viewed them very negatively (Toscani et al 1991). Two reasons were posited for this: increasing secularization and thus disappearance of any belief in an afterlife, and an increasingly higher standard of living, the philosophy of which consists of 'leading a full life'. Bryant (1991) defended this last suggestion by arguing that:

Our fascination for things and power makes us ill prepared to face death . . . (since) it causes us to devalue what might provide the greatest comfort (in dying): . . . honest, loving relationships and faith in God.

Bryant is a chaplain and therefore his statement could elicit controversy but with or without faith, he does have a point. In a study of constructions of death among the intrinsically religious it was concluded that such people have already solved their personal existential problem and look for a life after this one; thus, their level of 'death concern' was significantly lower ($p = < 0.001$) (Powell & Thorson 1991).

It has been shown that facing death is a time when patients may consider where their beliefs, if any, lie and may make changes in them, as in the case of a form of bargaining. It is also possible that, in the course of anger, people with religious beliefs may start to question them as they wonder if this is divine punishment or, as one person with cystic fibrosis stated:

It didn't seem fair. Why were so many patients dying? Why did the disease attack only children and young adults, giving them so little time to live? Why didn't the God of all creation intervene as another cystic struggled to breathe, infection raged wild inside his lungs, and the doctors watched helplessly? (Williman 1988).

When it comes to spiritual care, nurses still seem to think it is only a job for the chaplain and only at a time of crisis. Rhodes & Carlisle (1990) believe that it is better to involve the chaplain before imminent death.

No solid guidelines for specific interventions for nurses have been found that are specific to working with the terminally ill. However, the need for spiritual care and support for terminally ill patients has been recognized by the WHO (Anstey 1993), by the working group of representatives from the RCN Hospice Nurse Managers Forum and the Palliative Nursing Care Group (Beattie 1993). It would appear, therefore, that the interventions suggested earlier should also be relevant in the care of the dying patient, though with consideration of the spiritual problems that are particular to this client group. It has also been documented that nurses working with the terminally ill are also at risk from spiritual pain, as a consequence of their work 'taking its toll' (Rhodes & Carlisle 1990, Clark 1991). A good staff support network is recommended, where members can talk, share, laugh or cry together (Clark 1991).

WHAT HAS BEEN ACHIEVED?

Am I going round in circles or dare I hope I am on a spiral? But if a spiral, am I going up or down it? (Lewis 1966).

What conclusions, if any, can be drawn from the literature which has been studied? Are we any nearer to some answers? Or are we doomed to go on thinking that spirituality is a mystical concept which seems so vital, yet so user-unfriendly?

Should all nurses now enrol on counselling courses, whilst studying degrees in theology and philosophy, before attempting to approach the patient in the name of spirituality? Curtis (1983, cited in Copp 1986) studied the role of the nurse as patient advocate. Her discovery seems also applicable to spirituality:

I found the nurse (as patient advocate) depicted as a combination lawyer-theologian-psychologist-family counsellor and dragon slayer wrapped up in a white uniform. I might add that an ordinary mortal like me felt depressed, even oppressed, by this vision of supernurse.

However, it also seems that nurses have been unconsciously giving spiritual care for years (Morrison 1992). A metaanalysis of 19th and 20th century literature showed that nurses have always been very good at the practical care of the dying (Wolf 1991). Maybe all that is needed is for nurses to update their knowledge and understanding of the spiritual needs of patients in such a diverse society and to improve their counselling and communication skills. Because this is such a highly individual and personal area, the patients themselves will teach us more than any textbook or research paper. Maybe this is why there are still so many inconsistencies and so few conclusions in past research.

The following points have been concluded from this literature review:

1. Spirituality is a highly individual and personal area, which makes it a difficult subject to 'nail down' and fit into an all-encompassing definition.
2. Future research should perhaps concentrate more on how to find out what spirituality means to the patient and how to plan and give appropriate spiritual care to that patient.
3. Spiritual care involves simple, yet extremely important nursing skills and interventions, such as the ability to listen and give attention, to show that 'I really do care'. Morrison (1992) believes that spiritual care is: '. . . a normal, human activity, which takes place at various levels. Anything from a "hello" to a hug, from hand holding to a massage, from a sympathetic grunt to a prayer'.
4. Spiritual care should involve a multidisciplinary approach, where its members know who to involve and when. Murray (1991) suggested that training of professionals in the care of the dying might include a closer understanding of allies in the care of the whole person.

Some aspects of spirituality have not been explored. These include an overview of cultural and religious practices which nurses need to be aware of because of special diets, rituals and laws which may have a dramatic effect on care given and treatment plan. For instance, most people are familiar with the forbidden use of blood products for a Jehovah's Witness but there are so many other considerations for cultural practices, such as not giving a vegetarian Hindu a plate on which meat has been served (Green 1993), that whole chapters could be written on such measures alone.

The importance of the spiritual care of nurses themselves has also only briefly been mentioned. This is partly due to a lack of literature on the subject. Nurses need to ensure that their own spiritual needs are being met so that they do not plummet into spiritual distress, taking the patient with them. Spiritual care can be emotionally exhausting if the nurse is left to carry the burdens of patients with no-one to share, laugh or cry with. We must be careful not to produce another source of burnout in nursing.

Anthony-Salladay & McDonnell (1989) concluded from their study of spiritual care, ethical choices and patient advocacy that:

Perhaps more frequently, however, it is a quiet, private function of support and intuition as patients seek to come to a personal awareness of the meaning of illness. Advocacy (or indeed, spiritual care) exhibits a sensitivity to personal values, hopes and even unspoken prayer that shape an atmosphere of caring (p 549).

APPENDIX I SPIRITUAL HEALTH CONCERNS
(Morrison 1989 p 29)

Self
Acceptance of whole self
Gratitude for self
Care of body, mind and spirit
Growth of awareness
Sensitivity
Creative use of gifts
Acceptance/Use of defects and limitations
Sense of proportion and humour
Mortality

Creation
Responsibility for world
Taking of things as they are as starting point
Gratitude for creation
Awareness of interdependence

Others
Sense of responsibility
Care of others (in balance with care of self)
Differences not just tolerated, but enjoyed
Hostility ('You can't win them all')
Use of conflict
Contributing to healthy community

Life
Appreciation of life as it is
Meaning of life

Own purpose
Acceptance of conflict
Acceptance of suffering
Acceptance of tragedy
Acceptance of decay
Embracing change

REFERENCES

Ackerman M H, Henry M B, Graham K M, Coffey N 1993 Humor won, humor too: a model to incorporate humor into the health care setting. Nursing Forum 28(4): 9–16

American Holistic Nurses' Association 1992 code of ethics for holistic nurses. Journal of Holistic Nursing 10(3): 275–276

Anstey S 1993 Care in acute hospital units. Nursing Standard 7(19): 51

Anthony-Salladay S, McDonnell M M 1989 Spiritual care, ethical choices, and patient advocacy. Nursing Clinics of North America 24(2): 543–549

Austin D, Lennings C J 1993 Grief and religious belief: does belief moderate depression? Death Studies 17: 487–496

Barriball K L, While A 1994 Collecting data using a semi-structured interview: a discussion paper. Journal of Advanced Nursing 19: 328–335

Beattie R 1993 Standard setting in palliative care. Nursing Standard 7(19): 53

Bolund C 1993 Loss, mourning and growth in the process of dying. Palliative Medicine 7(2): 17–25

Bryant C 1991 Said another way. Nursing Forum 26(4): 31–34

Burnard P 1986 Picking up the pieces. Nursing Times 82(17): 37–39

Burnard P 1987 Spiritual distress and the nursing response: theoretical considerations and counselling skills. Journal of Advanced Nursing 12: 377–382

Burnard P 1988a Searching for meaning. Nursing Times 84(37): 34–36

Burnard P 1988b Coping with other people's emotions. Professional Nurse 4(1): 11–14

Burnard P 1988c Discussing spiritual issues with clients. Health Visitor 61: 371–372

Burnard P 1988d The spiritual needs of atheists and agnostics. Professional Nurse 4(3): 130–132

Burnard P 1990 Learning human skills, 2nd edn. Heinemann, Oxford

Canis P 1992 Attending the spirit. Nursing Times 88(32): 50

Chapman R 1974 The cry of the spirit. SCM, Gateshead

Charnes L S, Moore P S 1992 Meeting patients' spiritual needs: the Jewish perspective. Holistic Nursing Practice 6(3): 64–72

Clark B 1991 Spirituality in the hospice setting. Palliative Medicine 5(2): 151–154

Clark C C, Cross J R, Deane D M, Lowry L W 1991 Spirituality: integral to quality care. Holistic Nursing Practice 5(3): 67–76

Cole E J 1993 The near death experience. Intensive and Critical Care Nursing 9: 157–161

Colter J 1994 God's mechanic. Nursing 24(1): 41

Coon D 1988 Essentials of psychology – exploration and application, 4th edn. West, St Paul

Copp G, Dunn V 1993 Frequent and difficult problems perceived by nurses caring for the dying in community, hospice and acute care settings. Palliative Medicine 7(1): 19–25

Copp L A 1986 The nurse as advocate for vulnerable persons. Journal of Advanced Nursing 11: 255–263

Cumming A 1993 Patients' access to hospital chaplains. Nursing Standard 8(13/14): 30–31

Dickinson C 1975 The search for spiritual meaning. American Journal of Nursing 75(10): 1789–1793

Forbis P A 1988 Meeting patients' spiritual needs. Geriatric Nursing 9(3): 158–159

Fromm E 1961 Marx's concept of man. Ungar, New York

Fromm E, Xirau R 1968 The nature of man. Collier Macmillan, London

Garrett G 1991 A natural way to go? Professional Nurse 6(12): 744–749

Green J 1991 Death with dignity. Nursing Times/Macmillan, London

Green J 1993 Death with dignity: volume II. Nursing Times/Macmillan, London

Greyson B 1992 Reduced death threat in near death experiencers. Death Studies 16: 523–536

Hampe S O 1975 Needs of the grieving spouse in a hospital setting. Nursing Research 24(2): 113–119

Harrison J, Burnard P 1993 Spirituality and nursing practice. Avebury, Aldershot

Hegarty P 1991 The prayer. Nursing Times 87(36): 30

Heriot C S 1992 Spirituality and ageing. Holistic Nursing Practice 7(1): 22–31

Heron J 1990 Helping the client. Sage, London

Herth K 1990 Fostering hope in terminally ill people. Journal of Advanced Nursing 15: 1250–1259

Highfield M F 1992 Spiritual health of oncology patients: nurse and patient perspectives. Cancer Nursing 15(1): 1–8

Holy Bible. New King James Version (1990) Thomas Nelson, Nashville

International Council of Nurses 1973 Code for nurses. Imprimeries Populaires, Geneva

Jasper M A 1994 Issues in phenomenology for researchers of nursing. Journal of Advanced Nursing 19: 306–314

Kim M J, McFarland G K, McLane A M 1991 Pocket guide to nursing diagnoses, 4th edn. Mosby Year Book, St Louis

Kübler-Ross E 1970 On death and dying. Tavistock/Routledge, London

Labun E 1988 Spiritual care: an element in nursing care planning. Journal of Advanced Nursing 13: 314–320

Lewis C S 1966 A grief observed. Faber and Faber, London

Loader S 1990 Heaven can wait. Professional Nurse 5(9): 458–463

Mickley J R, Soeken K, Belcher A 1992 Spiritual well-being, religiousness and hope among women with breast cancer. IMAGE: Journal of Nursing Scholarship 24(4): 267–272

Misiak H, Sexton V S 1973 Phenomenological, existential and humanistic psychologies: a historical survey. Grone & Stratton, London

Morrison R 1989 Spiritual health care and the nurse. Nursing Standard 4(13/14): 28–29

Morrison R 1990a Spiritual health care and the nurse. Nursing Standard 4(36): 32–34

Morrison R 1990b Spiritual health care and the nurse. Nursing Standard 5(5): 34–35

Morrison R 1992 Diagnosing spiritual pain in patients. Nursing Standard 6(25): 36–38

Murray D B 1991 Attitudes and perceptions affecting Scottish clergy in their care of the dying. Palliative Medicine 5(3): 233–236

O'Connor A P, Wicker C A, Germino B B 1990 Understanding the cancer patient's search for meaning. Cancer Nursing 13(3): 167–175

Ozinga J R 1991 Communism – the story of the idea and its implementation, 2nd edn. Prentice Hall, New Jersey

Parse R R, Coyne A B, Smith M J 1985 Nursing research: qualitative methods. Brady, Maryland

Pierce J D, Hutton E 1992 Applying the concepts of the Neuman systems model. Nursing Forum 27(1): 15–18

Polanyi M 1962 Personal knowledge. University of Chicago Press, Chicago

Powell F C, Thorson J A 1991 Constructions of death among those high in intrinsic religious motivation: a factor analytic study. Death Studies 15: 131–138

Quesenberry L, Rittman M R 1993 When other words fail. American Journal of Nursing 93(3): 120

Reed J 1994 Phenomenology without phenomena: a discussion of the use of phenomenology to examine expertise in long term care of elderly patients. Journal of Advanced Nursing 19: 336–341

Rew L, Shirejian P 1993 Sexually abused adolescent: conceptualisation of sexual trauma and nursing interventions. Journal of Psychosocial Nursing 31(12): 29–33

Rhodes A, Carlisle D 1990 Spiritual services. Nursing Times 86(50): 30–31

Richards S H 1994 Finding the means to carry on: suicidal feeling in cancer patients. Professional Nurse 9(5): 334–339

Robbins C 1991 Body, mind and spirit. Nursing 4(31): 9–11

Schneider S, Kastenbaum R 1993 Patterns and meanings of prayer in hospice caregivers: an exploratory study. Death Studies 17: 471–485

Simsen B 1988 Nursing the spirit. Nursing Times 84(37): 31–33

Speck P 1992 Nursing the soul. Nursing Times 88(23): 22

Taylor P B, Ferszt G G 1994 Letting go of a loved one. Nursing 24(1): 55–56

Thompson J 1990 A chaplain's personal view of intensive care. Intensive Care Nursing 6: 192–195

Toscani F, Cantoni L, DiMola G, Mori M, Santosuasso A, Tamburini M 1991 Death and dying: perceptions and attitudes in Italy. Palliative Medicine 5(4): 334–343

UKCC 1992 Code of professional conduct, 3rd edn. UKCC, London

Webber J 1993 A specialised role in the health care setting. Nursing Standard 7(19): 52–53

Williman A 1988 The pain and gain of suffering. HiCall 67(3): Part 5, 6–8

Wolf Z R 1991 Care of dying patients and patients after death: patterns of care in nursing history. Death Studies 15: 81–93

Wyatt P 1993 The role of nurses in counselling the terminally ill patient. British Journal of Nursing 2(14): 701–704

FURTHER READING

Allen C 1991 The inner light. Nursing Standard 5(20): 52–53

Benner P, Wrubel J 1989 The primacy of caring: stress and coping in health and illness. Addison-Wesley, California

Frankl V 1962 Man's search for meaning. Hodder and Stoughton, Sevenoaks

Hasler K 1993 Bereavement counselling (continuing education series: article 306). Nursing Standard 7(4): 31–34

Jay P 1990 Relatives caring for the terminally ill. Nursing Standard 5(5): 30–32

Kapp M B 1993 Living and dying the Jewish way: secular rights and religious duties. Death Studies 17: 267–276

Marks M 1993 Palliative care: learning unit 002 (RCN nursing update). Nursing Standard 8(2): 1–8

Olson M 1992 Near death experiences and the elderly. Holistic Nursing Practice 7(1): 16–21

Sharma D L 1990 Hindu attitude toward suffering, dying and death. Palliative Medicine 4(3): 235–238

Short R L 1990 The Bible according to Peanuts. Collins Fount, London

Singh Sambhi P, Cole W O 1990 Caring for Sikh patients. Palliative Medicine 4(3): 229–233

Swaffield L 1988 Religious roots. Nursing Times 84(37): 28–29

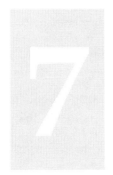

The most significant 'nothing': a concept analysis of personal space

Karen Poole

Commentary

In writing this chapter, Karen Poole has comprehensively explored an area that should be at the forefront of every nurse's concern, whether working in the community or hospital setting. Despite this, in choosing the subject, Karen identified an area that has only recently received attention from the nursing community. It is a concept that has for many years received much attention from the field of environmental psychology but, as the chapter will show, it is still an area that has considerable scope for research from a nursing perspective.

But this work represents much more than just an exploration of personal space. Karen chose to reflect a current trend in nursing by not trying to create an all-encompassing theory of personal space, preferring to follow the process of concept analysis.

In order to achieve this Karen adopted Rodgers' (1989) framework for concept analysis, exploring and bringing together into a coherent whole a very wide range of literature, from the fields of anthropology, environmental psychology and ethology or animal psychology, sociology and of course nursing.

Read this chapter if you would like to find out about personal space and its significance for nursing practice but also read it if you would like to find out how to perform a concept analysis. Finally, the contents of this chapter represent an excellent example of how to achieve a high level of critical analysis and synthesis of pertinent literature.

Some thirty inches from my nose
The frontier of my person goes,
And all of the untilled air between
Is private pagus or demesne.
Stranger, unless with bedroom eyes
I beckon you to fraternise,
Beware of rudely crossing it;
I have no gun, but I can spit.

(W H Auden 1965)

ABSTRACT

Throughout the 20th century social scientists have been interested in how organisms use space. Each of us possesses a private and personal area that regulates the distance at which we interact. This space has been regarded as the most 'significant nothing', that affects all interpersonal interactions (Pluckhan 1968).

The concept of personal space has intrigued environmental psychologists for decades, but it is only in more recent years that nurse researchers have addressed this phenomenon.

The inconsistencies and confusion surrounding the nature of personal space has prompted the adoption of Rodgers' (1989) concept analysis framework as a strategy to guide and structure this literature review. A systematic use of this 'evolutionary' approach led to the construction of a conceptual definition of personal space. The review addresses the nature of the concept and its implications for nursing practice. The analysis culminates in the presentation of a model case to illustrate personal space and concludes by identifying further research questions and recommendations for the nursing profession.

INTRODUCTION

In the midst of an animated conversation the person with whom you are talking shuffles closer towards you. You are able to see the loose hair coiled upon the threads of her woollen sweater, the smudge of lipstick on her tooth, you can smell the trace of stale coffee on her warm breath. Their proximity is overbearing, so you surreptitiously edge backwards, increasing the distance between yourself and this other person. Again they creep forward, once more you retreat. To the observer it is a *pas de deux*, yet why do those few inches matter, why do you feel such discomfort?

Imagine lying in a bed, an alien clinical hospital bed, a rigid counterpane masking stiff starched sheets. You are unable to move without assistance. A young nurse approaches clutching a long grey metallic box. The nurse picks up the documents from the wired basket hanging from your bed and proceeds to sit next to you, denting your bed linen. His name badge is now clearly visible, the stain of pink hand wash on his white expanse obvious. This stranger is close, too close, but you cannot move away.

The 'proxemic' dance (Hall 1966) is brought to a halt.

Personal space is that area immediately surrounding each of us that we consider exclusively ours. It is a subject rarely discussed, but it is present in all our interactions. How often have you heard the expressions 'I keep her at arm's length', 'She was breathing down my neck' or 'I wouldn't touch him with a 10 foot barge pole'? So-called 'distance phrases' (Altman & Chemers 1989) are very much part of our common language. These phrases illustrate the simple but often unverbalized fact that we actively use distance between ourselves and others in everyday relationships.

The relationship between a patient and a nurse is unique. Complete strangers (frequently of different generations) interact in very close proximity more usually associated with those of intimate acquaintance. An intrusion of personal space is inevitable. How is such trespassing tolerated? Is it legitimized by the perceived roles of health professionals? These questions and many more are unearthed as the concept of personal space is addressed.

CONCEPT ANALYSIS

It has been stated that the discipline of nursing is engaged in the quest to develop a knowledge base (Meleis 1991, Norris 1982, Rodgers 1989). In recent years, there has been an increasing concern with concepts and the resolution of conceptual problems as a component of intellectual advancement and concept analysis has emerged as an important means of examining common phenomena (Wuest 1994).

The concept of personal space has been a neglected area of concern within nursing research. The paucity of nursing studies and the plethora of experiments by environmental psychologists have resulted in much confusion and inconsistency in defining the nature and characteristics of personal space. Evans & Howard (1973), in a review of environmental psychology investigations of spatial behaviour research, stated:

Piecemeal examination of individual variables based upon a single dependent measure will continue to provide us with much data and little insight into the nature of personal space.

It is for this reason that concept analysis has been adopted to structure this literature review and organize the material, whilst simultaneously clarifying the concept and illustrating its significance in nursing practice.

There are numerous definitions of concepts, but the explanation most frequently cited is that offered by Hardy (1974) who stated that 'Concepts are mental images about an action or a thing' (p 145). Implicit in this definition is the observation that concepts are not the things or actions themselves but simply the construct or image in the mind. Therefore, concepts are inevitably tinted by the theorist's perception, experience and philosophical orientation.

Concepts and meaning are very closely related; indeed, the process of forming a concept and learning the meaning of a word are often one and the same. Words and other semantic symbols acquire a meaning that has been socially constructed by our heritage and will thus change throughout time, culture and context. Rodgers (1989) develops this idea to describe a dynamic cyclical process of concept development which is affected by three influences, namely significance, use and application.

An analysis of any concept will by its very nature be time, culture and context specific. Concepts are recognized as the basic elements of theory, the basis from which interrelationships and hypotheses are made. Just like the construction of any building, it is imperative that the foundation theories are structurally sound. The process recommended by Wilson (1963) to ensure this stability is concept analysis. This has been defined by Walker & Avant (1988) as '. . . a formal linguistic procedure to determine the essential attributes of concepts' (p 35).

Wilson (1963) is frequently credited as the innovator of concept analysis. He described the notion at length, highlighting the shift of intellectual enquiry required to think with concepts. Wilson did not present a sequential framework within which analysis is to occur, he merely suggested a series of techniques designed to assist in the creative process of concept clarification. These techniques were organized into a framework by Walker & Avant (1988 p 37) and are as follows:

1. Select a concept.
2. Determine the aims and purposes of analysis.
3. Identify all possible uses of the concept.
4. Determine the defining attributes.
5. Construct a model case.
6. Construct borderline, related, contrary, invented and illegitimate cases.
7. Identify antecedents and consequences.
8. Define empirical referents.

The framework encourages the investigator to examine all possible uses of the concept under review, drawing upon literature from a multitude of disciplines. From this rich database, those attributes that consistently appear are important in determining the critical dimensions of the concept. The analysis results in a precise operational definition and forms a common reference point for nursing practice (Chinn & Kramer 1991). The most pertinent limitation of the process is that the quality of any analysis is directly proportional to the analytical ability of the investigator. For this reason, Walker & Avant (1988) comment that regardless of how rigorous the analysis, the end product must always be tentatively concluded.

Concept analysis frameworks have traditionally been regarded as intrinsic to the process of literature review, clarifying the concepts that are used in hypothesis generation. Despite the emergence of new methods of concept analysis, for example the hybrid model proposed by Schwartz-Barcott & Kim (1986) and simultaneous concept analysis devised by Haase et al (1992), there has been a concerning unquestioning acceptance of Walker & Avant's framework. The implications and philosophical foundations of conducting an analysis of a concept were frequently ignored until Rodgers (1989) highlighted these deficits in her 'evolutionary' approach to analysis and further incongruencies were discussed by Wuest (1994).

In exploring the philosophical basis of concepts, Rodgers describes two primary schools of thought, referred to as the 'entity' and 'disposition' views. Entity views regard a concept as a 'thing' such as an image, idea, word or element in a system of logic. In contrast, dispositional views perceive concepts as habits, abilities to perform behaviours or the capacity for word use (Rodgers 1989).

Traditional approaches to analysis, such as the framework proposed by Walker & Avant (1988), have been founded in the entity school of thought, focusing upon the isolation of a concept with rigid defined boundaries. The reductionist objective view of reality results in the static description of a concept as a mirror of reality and fails to acknowledge its inherent social construction (Chinn & Kramer 1991). In recognition of the coexistence and interrelationships between concepts, Rodgers (1989) introduces her evolutionary approach to analysis rooted from a 'dispositional stance'.

It could be proposed that Rodgers merely highlights the thoughts and views originally expressed by Wilson (1963), but she makes an invaluable contribution in outlining her revised approach to concept analysis, producing the following framework:

1. Identify and name the concept of interest.
2. Identify the surrogate terms and relevant uses of the concept.
3. Identify and select an appropriate realm for data collection.
4. Identify the attributes.
5. Identify the referents, antecedents and consequences.

6. Identify concepts related to the concept of interest.
7. Identify a model case of the concept.

Attention is directed towards the recognition of surrogate terms. Individual concepts may be employed in association with several different terms or several terms may operate as manifestations of the concept. In Walker & Avant's (1988) framework, illegitimate cases of the concept were frequently constructed, exploiting conflict of terminology rather than concepts.

The evolutionary approach values wholeness, dynamism and interconnectivity and therefore has a substantial utility value for nursing. Rodgers herself omits to conduct an analysis of a concept according to her approach; however, this does not appear to have deterred other researchers from using the framework, for example Gibson (1991), Teasdale (1989) and Attree (1993).

Emanating from a feminist perspective, Wuest (1994) explores the incongruencies between the philosophical underpinnings of concept analysis and feminist inquiry. Internal incompatibilities include problems with validation, generalizability and measurement. Wuest (1994) maintains that a concept can only be validated through dialogue with those experiencing the concept and therefore concept analysis should not simply be an individual scholarly pursuit. Furthermore, the development of model cases is problematic because universalization may make the concept unrecognizable at an individual level. Similarly, conventional instruments devised from universal criteria are regarded as failing to capture the depth and breadth of women's lived experiences and thus the identification of empirical referents for a given concept is troublesome. Nevertheless, Wuest (1994) concludes that these incongruencies are not insurmountable and a feminist approach to concept analysis can reveal the social construction of a concept and the gender, racial and class bias inherent in it.

The process of concept analysis is not without its difficulties. Wilson (1963) identified the feelings of being hopelessly lost, a tendency to moralize, a compulsion to analyse everything and a disposition to engage in superficial fluency. However, Kemp (1985) maintains that the process of concept analysis enhances critical thinking and stimulates creative imaginative writing. It is a means of amalgamating information from a multitude of disciplines, introducing a richness of perspectives. Not least, it reduces ambiguity and vagueness of concepts fundamental to practice.

The structured framework of concept analysis is an ideal means of handling data in a subject that has previously been inadequately addressed, such as personal space, hence the adoption of Rodgers' evolutionary approach to guide the development of this literature review. Minor revisions have been made to the framework, notably the omission of the identification of an appropriate realm for data collection. Whilst systematic sampling increases the rigour of the analysis, the nature of this investigation does not dictate a need for detailed documentation. In a move to negate the accusation that concept analyses frequently degenerate into 'academic exercises' (Diers 1991), an additional stage has been introduced to this framework. This stage, 'the identification of implications for nursing', is also congruent with Rodgers' evolutionary focus of applicability and interconnectivity.

IDENTIFICATION OF THE CONCEPT OF INTEREST

We treat space somewhat as we treat sex. It is there but we don't talk about it (Hall 1966).

One only has to walk into the local newsagent and glance at the tabloid press and glossy magazines to see that sex is talked about and, more to the point, sex sells. Hardly the same can be said of space. Yet space has not been completely overlooked. Amidst all the glamour and gossip the term 'personal space' has been murmured.

In an article captioned 'Space Invaders', Jane Alexander (1993) of the *Daily Mail* asks of the readers 'Was Richard Branson's glad handling of Princess Diana just a touch too much?'. A photograph shows a distinctly uncomfortable Princess with the exuberant entrepreneur, fuelling a discussion of the concept of personal space, a concept that, according to the nameless scientists and researchers, will unlock the secrets to avoiding 'misunderstandings, embarrassment and any number of social *faux pas*'.

One can understand why such a topic should be of interest. People will go to great lengths to avoid intruding upon the interaction space of others and are quite uncomfortable when they cannot help but do so.

Space has been defined as 'room to move about' and 'room to put our bodies in' (Pluckhan 1968). Space is a non-entity, but within a relationship it has the power to convey meaning. Indeed, as Pluckhan (1968) herself stated, 'It is undoubtedly the most significant "nothing" which affects our intrapersonal and interpersonal communication'.

Such a phenomenon is readily observable on entering a closed space, such as a lift. After manoeuvring into the metallic box, the appropriate button is pressed and a position hastily secured.

Even if there is only one other person in the vicinity, the distance between them is as large as practically possible. Eye contact is eliminated as if it is a prerequisite for entry, gaze focuses on the floor indicator or alternatively on the ground. Conversation ceases upon entry to the lift and resumes upon leaving. This non-interaction is attributable to the fact that passengers are forced to adopt unusually intimate interpersonal distances.

This phenomenon is not some new concept accompanying developing technology. Throughout the 20th century social scientists have been interested in how organisms utilize space. Early research into the area of human spatial behaviour was based primarily upon the work of ornithologists and ethologists observing the territorial behaviour and distance regulation of animals and birds. Hediger (1950, cited by Little 1965) has been identified (Aiello 1987) as the animal psychologist with greatest influence upon the early development of distance regulation patterns. Hediger described several distance zones that animals maintain from one another. Four such zones were the foundation for zones later constructed to interpret human interaction (Hall 1966).

Hediger also suggested the notion that each animal is surrounded by a series of bubbles and balloons that allow proper spacing between it and other animals, citing the common observation of birds evenly spaced along a telephone wire. This graphic analogy was transposed by von Uexkull (1957, cited by Sommer 1959) into a description of human beings existing in soap-bubble worlds.

In fact, Katz (1937, cited by Little 1965) has been credited as the first to coin the term 'personal space'. It is interesting to note his animated description of the concept as the shell of a snail. Whilst research into the area of human spatial behaviour does predate the 1960s it was during this decade that significant advances were made in the attention that social scientists paid to the topic. Many of the approaches to the concept of personal space were adapted from those frameworks relating to the consequences of inappropriate close spacing. Overstimulation models of arousal, stress and overload suggest that an individual maintains a preferred interaction distance from others.

It was E T Hall (1966), an anthropologist, who sensitized social and behavioural scientists to human spacing in his book *The Hidden Dimension*. Hall posited two key ideas in his work:

1. North Americans systematically use four distinct spatial zones in interactions with others.
2. Distinct cultures use different space as a communication vehicle in distinctive ways.

Hall went on to describe the term 'proxemics' to refer to:

... the study of how man unconsciously structures micro-space, the distance between men in the conduct of daily transactions, the organization of space in his houses and buildings and ultimately the layout of his towns.

Such influential work is further discussed in the next section. At that time, in another significant book entitled *Personal Space, the Behavioural Basis of Design* (Sommer 1969), spatial behaviour was examined as a series of experiments investigating individual variables influencing the use of space.

Parallel developments also began in many other disciplines such as sociology, ecology, psychiatry and architecture. Sadly, nursing was not one of these contributing disciplines, yet over recent years as nursing has embraced and incorporated knowledge from other areas, it has become implicit that the concept of personal space is fundamental to all interactions, not least those between the patient and the nurse.

SURROGATE TERMS AND RELEVANT USES

When a concept analysis is conducted in a linguistic manner, Rodgers (1989) proposes that it is necessary to identify surrogate terms in order to determine those synonyms used to convey the concept.

As with many other concepts, the term 'personal space' has been subject to misunderstanding and inappropriate use. A history of contributions from a multitude of disciplines has resulted in an abundance of terms that have been used interchangeably with significant consequences. The majority of extensive research studies have been conducted within the field of environmental psychology. The term 'personal space' has become the label most often used to refer to the whole realm of human spatial behaviour. In addition, there are numerous terms that have also become synonymous with 'personal space' – for example, 'personal territory', 'personal distance' and 'personal boundaries'. Having evolved from strong ethological tradition and a focus upon territorial behaviour, these surrogate terms have coexisted and frequently overlapped until an eminent researcher has distinguished one from another, for example, Sommer (1959).

The difficulty arises on trying to identify a true surrogate term as distinct from a separate but related concept. As no universally accepted definition of personal space has ever been developed, the distinction is purely subjective and somewhat arbitrary.

Confusion with 'personal territory' most probably stems from early definitions of territorial behaviour. Ardery (1966) used the term to describe the inward compulsion in an animate being to possess and defend a space. Such a proposition clearly has elements congruent with features commonly associated with personal space. Nevertheless, Little (1985) presented a comprehensive rationale identifying territory as a separate but related concept to personal space. The defining characteristics will be utilized in the identification of attributes.

Aiello (1987) describes personal space as a dichotomous concept with two distinct functions. The first is the protective aspect of personal space, an observation that can be undoubtedly linked to territorial behaviour. Secondly, personal space has a more active component: communication.

As previously mentioned, the most prominent researcher to theorize about the active use of space was E T Hall (1966). In his book *The Hidden Dimension*, Hall describes a study of man's use of space as a vehicle of communication, in which people manipulate interactional distances in order to attain desired levels of involvement. Hall classifies four spatial zones, each with a near and far phase, that reflect four principal categories of relationships and the types of activities and spaces corresponding to them.

The intimate zone 0–1.5 ft

At a specified near distance of zero to 0.5 ft and a far phase to 1.5 ft, this distance allows activities with possible body contact. It provides the medium within which a number of communication channels operate. Heat, olfactory cues, visual cues and auditory cues are highly significant, slight changes being immediately detectable. Individuals interacting in this distance zone are usually on close terms. Such interaction with other persons is seen as inappropriate and creates tension and stress.

The personal zone 1.5–4 ft

The personal zone (with a near phase of 1.5–2.4 ft and a far phase of 2.4–4 ft) is that frequently identified by researchers as a definition of personal space (Allekian 1973, Lane 1989). It is hypothesized that movement beyond 4 ft is associated with a threat to control and is therefore accompanied by an increase in anxiety. At this distance the communication cues still remain rich.

The social zone 4–12 ft

Used in public, business and social settings, at this distance olfactory and heat cues are absent. The close phase is identified at a distance of 4–7 ft and the far phase at 7–12 ft. Touching is not possible and visual and auditory cues are the main vehicle of communication.

The public zone 12 ft and over

At distances of 12–25 ft and a far phase of 25 ft and over, this distance is only used between a speaker and an audience. Fine details are no longer visible and the accentuation of movements and enunciation of words are required in order to be understood.

Hall's spatial zones are frequently cited in the literature associated with personal space, but very rarely are his findings criticized. One notable exception is found in the work of the environmental psychologist Aiello (1987). There is no evidence to confirm that it is at the different zonal transition points that marked differences in the experience of interactants occur. Rather, these different experiences would change in conjunction with the gradual variance in sensory inputs. In addition, an infinite number of characteristics of the participants and their environment would make the classification of set distances very approximate at best. Although virtually never mentioned in the literature, Hall himself has noted that 'the measured distances vary somewhat with difference in personality and environmental factors' (p 116).

Hall's data were obtained through interviews and observations of middle-class healthy white North American adults. Today it could be assumed that as times and norms change, subjects may show slightly different behaviours. Various studies, however, confirm that Hall's model is applicable to other cultures, although the distances may vary within a predictable range (Altman & Chemers 1989).

Arguably it is Hall's spatial zone distances that have led to the adoption of the term 'interpersonal distance'. Most researchers utilize the terms 'personal space' and 'interpersonal distance' interchangeably (for example, Altman & Chemers 1989). Others, however, have distinguished between the two (Edney et al 1976) and have actually measured the two concepts independently.

It could be proposed that personal distance is in fact a component of personal space. Sommer (1959) stated: '. . . personal distance is the distance that the organism customarily places between itself and other organisms'. When this is compared with the description of personal space offered by Little (1959): '. . . the area immediately surrounding the person in which the majority of his interactions take place', it is apparent that distance is perhaps a measurement of the personal space. As defining attributes of the concept are addressed this idea will be reinforced.

Almost inherent in the discussion of territory and spatial distances is the notion of boundaries. As Knowles (1980, cited by Aiello 1987) stated, 'One is either in or out of your personal space'. Such a statement presupposes the crossing of a boundary, distinct from the transition of one zone to another. Altman & Chemers (1989) regard the space around a person's body as an 'ultimate barrier' that can be used to make oneself more or less accessible to another human being. The degree to which a boundary is permeable or flexible is dependent upon individuals and their perceptions of the environment as safe or threatening (Scott 1988).

General systems theorists, for example Miller (1973), Rogers (1970) and Auger (1976), have incorporated boundaries into their conceptual frameworks of nursing's perception of human life. Although recognizing that the notion of boundaries is utilized somewhat differently within each individual theory, Meisenhelder (1982) vividly concluded that:

Human defences are layered and can be compared to a castle; to penetrate the stone walls and gain access to the interior, one must first cross the moat.

Whatever model of nursing is used to deliver care, nurses must identify by what means they are going to negotiate such a stretch of water. Firstly, however, the nature of this 'moat' must be addressed by the filtering of terms in order to clarify the defining attributes of personal space.

ATTRIBUTES

In any concept analysis the determination of defining attributes is the most critical part of the process, forming the pivot from which all other inferences are made. Perhaps the most intellectually demanding section, it must be emphasized that the rigorous selection of characteristics unique to any concept is dependent upon the ability of the investigator. A critical review of previous definitions is instrumental in pinpointing idiosyncrasies that differentiate personal space from other similar related concepts. In other words, it could be stated that:

Like the porcupine in Schopenfauer's fable, people like to be close enough to obtain warmth and comradeship but far enough away to avoid pricking one another (Sommer 1959).

This depiction of personal space captures the essence of the concept, the very real experience of possessing a private area that regulates the distance at which people interact.

In a series of experiments, Felipe & Sommer (1966) identified students sitting alone at a table and sat within 12 inches of them, shoulder to shoulder. They consistently found that half the students left the room after 10 minutes and noted that students often used objects as barriers, including chairs to protect their space. Only one out of 80 students asked the experimenter to move, implying that personal space is an 'unspoken dimension', comparable to Pluckhan's (1968) 'space: the silent language'.

Sommer's further work on sociopetal (positions that encourage conversation) and sociofugal (positions that do not encourage interaction) seating arrangements illustrated the optimal positions for interaction in relationship to personal space. Following a preliminary observation of the quality and number of interactions among residents in the lounge of a nursing home, Sommer noted that residents seemed to be arranged by the positioning of the furniture. Upon rearranging the chairs from straight rows to corner to corner or face to face at a small table Sommer found, within two weeks, that interaction among the residents had doubled. Sommer attributed his results to the notion of personal space. The addition of tables offered tangible barriers and extra area to each resident's personal space. The table area legitimized personal articles such as books and handicrafts in the environment. Corner to corner seating not only allowed for eye contact, but gave more distance between individuals than rows.

From such findings it is implicit that personal space functions as an unconsciously marked territory. These distinguishing features include:

- Personal space is portable whereas territory is relatively stationary.
- The boundaries of personal space are invisible, whilst those of territory are usually marked.
- The person's body is the centre of his/her personal space, but not of his/her territory.
- If personal space is intruded the person tends to withdraw, if territory is intruded the person fights to defend (Sommer 1959).

These characteristic elements of personal space are tantamount to the first attempt to establish defining attributes and interestingly are widely used in subsequent literature.

The notion of portable personal space has captured the imagination of many writers and has been likened to a snail shell (Katz 1937, cited by Little 1965), a soap bubble (Von Uexkull 1957, cited by Sommer 1959) and an aura (Stern 1935, cited by Sommer 1959). Such images conjure up pictures of people walking around in some sort of giant transparent globe. All of these portrayals make the assumption that personal space is symmetrical in its dimensions, that it is finite in that it is edged by an invisible boundary.

Strube & Werner (1982) conducted a series of experiments in order to test their hypothesis that personal space would expand in response to potential loss of control (and therefore not be a defined size) and that the shape of personal space would be irregular. They explained to their 80 subjects that personal space was an 'area' or 'bubble' surrounding their body that was considered to belong exclusively to them. The subjects were given a ball of string and scissors to mark out the area that each felt to be exclusively theirs. The experiment progressed with a confederate adopting the role of a salesperson taking control and the subject the customer, who was told to resist buying the items. The results indicated that both interpersonal distances and claimed personal space were larger in the customer than the salesperson role, expanding in response to a perceived loss of control. Furthermore, the claimed personal space areas were not symmetrical in shape, but extruded to provide greatest defence where the threatening opponent was located.

Whilst these findings may be significant, one has to be aware that the data were collected with the subjects' knowledge, introducing an element of self-presentational or demand characteristic biases. It can also be questioned whether it is possible to translate an abstract subjective three-dimensional construct into a concrete two-dimensional observable measure. On comparison with other studies (such as Little 1965) it is reasonable to suggest that personal space does fluctuate in response to the environment and situation (a subject that is further explored later). For example, in contact sports, one's personal space contracts dramatically, but may extend to large areas in times of threat as when walking alone down a dark street.

In more recent years nurse researchers (Allekian 1987, Lane 1989) have investigated the notion of personal space. Despite recognizing in introductory explanations that personal space is a fluctuating, dynamic phenomenon, when actually defining the concept it is stipulated that: '. . . personal space extends outwards to a direction of four feet' (Lane 1989). If this definition is to be taken literally, personal space will be a circular area and hardly flexible. This distance of 4 feet has been lifted directly from Hall's (1966) work on spatial zones and whilst it is useful in determining the extent to which personal space might typically extend in a middle-class white North American, it ignores the subjectivity of the concept.

This criticism is reminiscent of Patterson's (1976) argument to 'burst' the personal space 'bubble', that conveys stability, when it has been shown that personal space boundaries change considerably according to setting, relationship and environment conditions (Little 1965).

Regardless of its size or shape, the personal space boundary marks one's separation from others. It could be suggested that in similar situations people have comparable personal space areas. One only has to look at the sideways shuffle along the curb when another person joins the bus queue, resulting in a spacing that replicates the previously mentioned birds on a telephone wire.

It has been suggested that the personal space boundary has an intrapersonal as well as an interpersonal function. The person's selection of what crosses the boundary establishes an identity and becomes a psychological part of the person (Simmel 1961, cited by Lyman & Scott 1967). As such, the significance of personal space cannot be underestimated.

Reflecting upon the wealth of definitions and explanations of the concept of personal space, there are several key features that have become inextricably associated with the concept, to the extent that they can be considered defining attributes. Those identified characteristics include:

- invisibility
- portability
- fluctuating boundary.

Therefore, personal space can be defined as the constant territorial claim of individuals to an invisible portable space surrounding their persons, enclosed by a boundary that fluctuates in response to certain variables.

ANTECEDENTS, CONSEQUENCES, REFERENTS

Antecedents are considered to be events or phenomena that precede an instance of the concept (Rodgers 1989). It is implicit in the notion of personal space that it is a perpetual reality, yet it is only evidenced when interactions occur. Indeed, personal space is only in existence because humans are social beings. That said, antecedents of personal space cannot be considered antecedents in the truest sense of the word; moreover, they are factors that have an impact upon personal space.

During the 1960s, there was a flurry of interest in those factors thought to influence personal space and a multitude of experiments were conducted by environmental psychologists to the extent that in a review of personal space literature, Aiello (1987) identified over 700 studies.

Approaching the concept of personal space from a nursing perspective through Rodgers' evolutionary view of concept analysis, it is difficult to embrace this highly reductionist investigation of antecedent factors. Nevertheless, the contribution that these studies have made in the creation of hypotheses regarding personal space cannot be disregarded. Altman (1975) identifies three broad categories within which the vast series of studies can be categorized:

1. Individual factors, including age, gender, culture, personality.
2. Interpersonal factors, including acquaintance, familiarity, social role.
3. Situational factors, including the effect of setting on the regulation of boundaries.

The majority of these studies have been conducted by environmental psychologists and have been comprehensively reviewed by Evans & Howard (1973) and Aiello (1987).

Before each of the three categories is discussed in turn, it is important to note that both or all participants in an interaction have these antecedents and they are not confined purely to the person who is being intruded upon.

Individual factors

Age is discussed first, because conflicting patterns of results involving other effects such as gender and culture are only unravelled when age is taken into account.

Personal space has been found to develop gradually and systematically as children grow older, interaction spaces being found to get larger and less variable from childhood to adolescence and stabilizing in middle adulthood (Mersels & Guardo 1969, cited in Evans & Howard 1973). Fry & Willis (1971) found that at the age of 8–10 years, children developed the capacity to elicit personal space invasion in others. The experiment involved the observation of adult reactions to children walking up to and standing 2–3 ft behind them whilst waiting in a queue. Arguably the experiment demonstrates little except adults' perceptions of appropriate contact with children of particular ages and nothing about personal space development in the children themselves.

Aiello (1987) suggests that human beings possess an inherent spatial mechanism and through the process of social learning involving imitation and reinforcement, children learn the accepted cultural pattern of proxemic behaviour. Thus, just as culture will influence the development of spatial behaviour, so will gender. In general, it has been suggested that females possess smaller personal space zones than men. This has been surmised from observations that during affiliation-focused interaction between women, interaction distances are smaller than those between men (Sommer 1959). However, in situations implying threat, this pattern has been seen to be reversed. In a laboratory-controlled study, McBride et al (1965) demonstrated that in North American female white subjects (aged between 19 and 23 years) their galvanic skin responses were greatest when approached by an experimenter of the opposite sex to a distance of 3 ft.

The size of personal space and the extent to which the boundaries are porous is also culture dependent. The major impetus for research into cultural variables was initiated by Hall (1966). Many studies have concentrated upon Hall's hypothesis of contact and non-contact cultures. Watson & Graves (1966, cited in Gifford 1987) observed discussion groups of North Americans and Arabs and found a greater degree of face to face orientation, closeness and touching in the Arabian group. South Americans, those from the Mediterranean and Arabs are generally acknowledged to be contact cultures, whereas the Scottish, Swedish and English are considered part of the non-contact culture. This is epitomized by George Mikes (1946), a Hungarian-born writer, who stated that: 'An Englishman, even if he is alone, forms an orderly queue of one' (p 44).

All persons from the same culture interact at a uniform distance in a given situation (Meisenhelder 1982). People therefore interpret another's spatial behaviour according to their own patterns; thus friendly actions may be misconstrued as aggressive threats.

Several researchers have looked at subcultures and mixed racial interactions within North Americans, but conflicting results have proved inconclusive.

Research studies assessing the influence of personality and psychological disorders were more abundant during the early years of spatial behaviour literature. Sommer (1959) reported that people with schizophrenia had an impaired sense of personal space and consistently intruded upon the personal space of those around them. Such an intrusion may cause the well person to draw away to maintain the customary personal space area, leaving the schizophrenic feeling rejected. It has been suggested (Aiello 1987) that one would expect the schizophrenic patient to have a larger than average personal space because of the need to withdraw from people and diminish sensory input, the dual functions of protection and communication being evident once again. It could be proposed that the schizophrenic has an adequate sense of personal space and the constant refining moves of others are a manifestation of negative labelling and stigmatism. This is substantiated by Kleck's (1969) findings that interaction distances with socially stigmatized individuals such as epileptics and the disabled were greatly increased.

Interpersonal factors

The relationship between individuals also has a strong effect upon their spatial behaviour. Interactions with those of a high degree of familiarity and acquaintance are often the most proximate. Little's (1965) findings support this. In a series of quasiprojective experiments, North American students positioned figurines according to a specified degree of acquaintance in a particular setting. In a further study, Little (1965) replaced the figures with live actors to justify the reliability of the projective technique. Both experiments demonstrated that the perceived interaction distances in a dyad were markedly influenced by the degree of acquaintance of the two members. If the pair were labelled as friends, they were seen as interacting at significantly closer distances than if termed acquaintances, with the label of strangers resulting in the greatest perceived distances. Nevertheless, the issue remains that the subject's perceived notions of acquaintance differences do not necessarily equate with reality, as a formerly unconscious phenomenon is brought under conscious scrutiny.

An unsolicited unwelcome intrusion into personal space is a perceived threat to identity and safety and is defended by gesture, posture or physical barriers (Meisenhelder 1982). The key to this defensive behaviour is said to be the human need to maintain complete control of one's space. The previously mentioned study by Strube & Werner (1982) illustrated the reactive increase in personal space to a perceived threat of loss of control. They concluded that claimed space will expand at closer distances when the close interpersonal distance is not chosen by the individual.

However, if there is no perceived loss of control there is no expansion in personal space. Once again, perception of loss of control will determine the ultimate reaction and in turn perception depends upon needs, experience, age, personality and culture (Allekian 1973). It could therefore be suggested that empowering an individual to maintain control will facilitate any necessary intrusions into his or her personal space.

Aiello (1987) maintains that we distance ourselves from those perceived as causing discomfort, anxiety and annoyance and move closer to those conveying warmth, comfort and strength. No referral is made to the victim who is unable to actually distance themselves. Sommer (1969) also suggests that those wishing to appear friendly or positive exhibit smaller personal space zones than others.

Situational factors

Individuals interact and encounter others not in a vacuum but in specific situational and environmental settings. Smaller, confining spaces increase interaction distance (Aiello 1987), a proposition confirmed by Little (1965) who found that perceived interaction distances increased progressively as dyads were moved from a street corner to a living room and finally to an office.

The societal and personal associations with any setting, such as a hospital, will also contribute to boundary fluctuation. Social roles and sickness are two factors that have been overlooked as variables for personal space and will be discussed later.

Aiello (1987) suggested that a more appropriate framework for classifying variables of personal space should have three dimensions:

1. perceived threat potential of invader;
2. perceived control potential of subject;
3. reason and circumstances surrounding invasion.

This framework is certainly more suitable for contextualizing the variables associated with the intrusions and invasions that occur between a hospitalized individual and a carer. In considering the antecedents of personal space, this very superficial overview has attempted to highlight the complexities of this phenomenon, demonstrating that the nature of personal space is a truly individualized affair, as Aiello (1987) concluded:

. . . importantly what makes any particular distance 'inappropriately close' is determined by all of the individual, relationship, situational and environmental factors (p 489).

CONSEQUENCES

Consequences follow an occurrence of the concept (Rodgers 1989). As previously stated, personal space is not an intermittent phenomenon, therefore consequences pertain to the maintenance or otherwise of personal space boundaries.

In the general conduct of everyday interactions we are continuously regulating our spatial behaviour in accordance with the fluctuation of personal space boundaries. It is inevitable that these boundaries will be compressed to the extent that they may even be crossed.

Consider rush hour on the London Underground. Salesmen, shoppers, students all sitting or standing, dictated by their steely surroundings, so many people in solitude. Personal spaces are severely compressed; is it really tiredness that prompts people to close their eyes? Each of those clutching at rails ensures that no part of their body or even their possessions are touching anyone else. If some misguided unbalanced individual does knock another, there is an instantaneous reflex, as their baggage is clutched closer to their body and a glaring glance is shot at the intruder.

This 'civil inattention' (Goffman 1963) and hostile reaction to personal space intrusion is typified in this description and has been synthesized for study in experimental conditions. The victims show signs of discomfort, embarrassment, restlessness, turning away or fidgeting, all of which are said to reflect attempts to increase the psychological distance between the victim and the intruder (Ingham 1978).

A considerable body of research-based knowledge on individual reactions to spatial invasion has been developed. Intrusion precipitates a stress response with measurable manifestations and these measurable responses have been used as indices in many studies, for example, behavioural reaction (Felipe & Sommer 1966), galvanic skin response (McBride et al 1965) and blood pressure (Hackworth 1976).

Apart from one notable exception, studies have overlooked the actual personal experience of the victims. Simmel (1961, cited by Lyman & Scott 1967) is the only investigator to acknowledge the lived experience of invasion. Simmel perceives personal space as an intellectual private property and an extension of the ego. Intrusion is regarded as a violation of the person and an exhibition of an extreme lack of respect. Nevertheless, no researcher has actually asked subjects to describe their feelings during the experience of personal space intrusion.

For Hall (1966), the distance at which one interacts with others is fully entwined with all other sensory modalities and determines the quality and quantity of stimuli exchanged. A series of mechanisms are used to regulate the level of contact between interactants and a number of studies have examined how interpersonal distance operates in conjunction with other behaviours such as eye contact, smiling and body posture. Three categories of models have been identified (Aiello 1987) that offer explanations for the relationship between spatial behaviour and verbal and non-verbal variables. These are the:

1. conflict/intimacy equilibrium models
2. arousal/attribution models
3. expectancy/discrepancy models.

Conflict/intimacy equilibrium models

Much of this work was stimulated by Argyle & Dean (1965). They proposed that people define an acceptable or appropriate level of intimacy they wish to maintain with another person. A blend of behaviours is used to achieve a state of equilibrium that reflects the desired level of intimacy. If people become more intimate than appropriate by either compressing or crossing personal space boundaries then behaviours operate in a compensatory fashion, for example by decreasing eye gaze. Thus, a state of equilibrium is restored. A review by Patterson (1976) found a reasonable level of support for this operation of compensatory mechanisms. However, there seem to be few studies examining the consequences of interactants being further away than is perceived necessary.

Arousal/attribution models

Patterson (1976) hypothesized that a change in someone's intimacy behaviour creates a state of arousal which is labelled either negative or positive. If positive there is reciprocity, if negative compensatory behaviour ensues.

Expectancy/discrepancy models

These models (Capella & Green 1982, Patterson 1982) attempt to encompass all possible outside variables that can affect the interactants' behaviour. Norms, situations, personality, relationships and, most significantly, social roles all contribute to expectancy.

Deviation from expected intimacy determines the behaviour of interactants; for example, if intimacy is greater than expected, the consequence is withdrawal.

This is particularly useful when considering the relationship between a patient and health professional and addresses the fact that the level of non-verbal interaction is not necessarily synonymous with the interactants' level of intimacy. The level of involvement may reflect nothing or very little about the social relationship.

It could be proposed that patients anticipate that nurses and physicians will adopt small interpersonal distances that intrude upon their personal space zone. This may be legitimized by the perceived role of such professionals and confirmed by the demarcation of status, including the wearing of uniform. Nevertheless, there are numerous variables accompanying hospitalization, not least of which are an alteration in health status, a relocation to a medical setting and a distancing from all who are familiar. To blindly impose any model of intrusion upon such a situation would be inappropriate, but the expectancy/attribution model does offer a means of embracing these variables when interpreting reactions to personal space intrusion.

REFERENTS

The purpose of identifying the referents of the concept is to clarify the range of events, situations or phenomena over which the application of a concept is considered to be appropriate (Rodgers 1989). Empirical referents themselves are: '. . . classes or categories of actual phenomena that by their existence or presence demonstrate the occurrence of the concept itself' (Walker & Avant 1988 p 40).

Having defined personal space as an invisible portable space edged by a fluctuating boundary, one can appreciate the difficulty of such a task. Generally, the majority of methods that have been created to study personal space have been designed to observe the behaviour of subjects, but not to understand their perceptions and experiences of body boundaries. Hall (1966) reasons that such an approach is justified and in fact desirable, stating that:

. . . proxemic patterns once learned are maintained largely out of conscious awareness and have to be investigated without resorting to prodding the minds of one's subjects . . . indeed, the very absence of conscious distortion is one of the principal reasons for investigating behaviour on this level (p 1003).

The literature shows three general approaches to the investigation of personal space: field/naturalistic techniques, simulation studies and laboratory methods. Field/naturalistic measures involve the direct and usually unobtrusive observation of naturally occurring interpersonal positioning in real settings. Sommer's (1959) study of students in libraries appears to be the first investigation of this kind. Minckley (1968), a recovery room nurse, utilized her position to conduct a field observation-led enquiry into the spatial awareness of 644 semiconscious patients recovering from surgical anaesthesia.

Simulation techniques, in contrast, actively engage the use of the subjects' conscious awareness. Real life is simulated on a model scale and subjects are required to position felt figures, line drawings, symbols or dolls as representatives of people according to their perception of interpersonal spacing. Extensively used by Little (1965), the technique has been widely criticized on the grounds of validity. This is because the exercise is dependent upon the memory of the subject and the subject's ability to transform actual distances to scaled-down distances.

Duke & Novicki (1972) presented a measure for interpersonal distance known as the Comfortable Interpersonal Distance (CID) scale. The scale required subjects to imagine themselves at the centre of eight radiating lines of 80 millimetres length and mark the distance at which they thought that they would feel uncomfortable with an approaching stimulus. Similar criticisms were levelled at this study, the only advantage being the ease of administering the scale.

Laboratory studies involve the actual distancing process between subjects within artificial laboratory conditions. The technique overcomes the model scale problems of simulation methods, but is still dependent upon the subjects' conscious awareness of spatial behaviour. Subjects are required to transform an 'out of awareness' process into one in which subjects are made very conscious of their distancing behaviour. It is no longer the 'hidden dimension', described by Hall (1966). Strube & Werner (1982) were criticized for the use of this methodology, where subjects were required to mark out their personal space zone with string.

Aiello (1987), however, cautions against completely rejecting simulation and laboratory methods of investigation, noting that there have been some differences among factors associated with personal space that have been reliably identified by all three types of measurement.

More recently, Lane (1989) developed a questionnaire to determine patients' and nurses' perceptions of personal space and territory intrusions. The Territorial Intrusion Personal Space

(TIPS) scale consisted of 14 randomly ordered concept statements, six representing territorial intrusions and eight personal space invasions. This approach circumnavigates all the problems of observing measurable interaction distance and focuses instead upon the lived experience of intrusion. Whilst it does bring the unconscious spatial mechanism into conscious use, rather than requiring the subject to demonstrate their personal space zones or territory, it directly establishes these facts by evaluating emotional reactions to various concept statements, for example, 'the nurse is sat upon your bed'. Arguably there is still a degree of simulation involved, because subjects are required to imagine the scenario and their reactions to it. However, this must surely be aided by their situational placing and frequent (although perhaps unconscious) experience of the action described.

As Evans & Howard (1973) stated:

... given the complex nature of human–environment variables exploration of personal space should employ a combination of techniques that seek to decrease bias and increase data generalizability.

RELATED CONCEPTS

In the process of researching the personal space literature, notions of privacy, territoriality and crowding frequently materialized and these terms can be regarded as separate but related concepts to personal space.

Privacy

Privacy is a widely used, all-encompassing term that seems to have eluded a consensus definition. Nevertheless, Altman (1975) is generally considered to have generated one of the most comprehensive distinctions when he stated that: 'Privacy is selective control of access to the self or to one's group' (p 18). As such, privacy has been regarded as a central construct around which other processes, including personal space and territorial behaviour, can be anchored. Thereby, personal space is assumed to be a regulatory mechanism by which an individual creates a desired level of openness or closedness to others.

Human beings are said to be social creatures, yet they constantly seek to achieve a state of privacy (Bauer 1993). This prompts the question, what are the functions of privacy? Westin (1967) offered four overlapping functions that are reminiscent of the dual functions of personal space, including personal autonomy, emotional release, self-evaluation and protected communication.

However, this is only one of many propositions (Altman 1975, Schwartz 1968) which are dependent upon the theory or model of privacy adopted.

There can be many forms of intrusion into one's privacy, be it physical intrusion into the personal space, unwanted publicity or disclosure of private information. In an exploratory study of patients' perceptions of their privacy in a German acute care hospital, Bauer (1993) found through the use of a Likert scale questionnaire that German patients were subjected to continuous violations of privacy during their stay. Patients' main concerns were fear of exposure of personal identity, fear of physical exposure, loss of personal autonomy and dependence on others. Bauer (1993) reported that aspects of personal space invasion and territorial intrusion were of secondary importance, control being the major determinant in the patients' perception of their privacy.

The ability to regulate and control privacy is hypothesized to be essential to people's well-being, viability and self-identity (Altman & Chemers 1989). These researchers depict territorial behaviour as one of several behavioural mechanisms that operate in the service of privacy, regulating access to the self.

Territoriality

Derived from its application to animal behaviour, human territoriality has been studied since the 1920s. Territoriality is the term used to describe the state which is characterized by possessiveness, control and authority over an area of physical space (Hayter 1981). It has been suggested by Roberts (1978, cited in Tungapalan 1982) that for the needs of territoriality to be fully met, the person must be in control of some space, able to establish rules for the space and to defend it against invasion and the right to do those things must be acknowledged by other persons.

There exist several theories of territoriality, some based on genetic heritage, others preferring learning as the determinant of behaviour. These theories, however, are controversial, speculative and mostly not research based (Gifford 1987).

Altman (1975) offers a distinct classification of territories as primary, secondary and public. This categorization seems to have superseded that originally proposed by Lyman & Scott (1967) of public, home, interactional and body territories. Primary territories are characterized by exclusive use and occupancy by a specific group or individual over an extended period of time, where access is rigidly controlled; Kerr (1985) uses physician's offices as an illustration. Secondary territories are less central to any one individual or group and are often shared with others by mutual consent, for example the nurses' station (Kerr 1985). Public territories are relatively temporary and readily accessible to almost anyone if they follow social norms and expectations of behaviour, for instance, hallways.

Clearly primary territories are the most private and have the most effective boundary control mechanisms. During hospitalization, however, patients are frequently situated in secondary territories and expected to perform behaviours (for example, sleeping, eating) that are usually performed in primary territories (Gifford 1987). It is for this reason that Hayter (1981) suggests it is important for nurses to obtain information about territorial needs when conducting the nursing assessment.

As with personal space, there are many variable factors that influence territoriality (Altman 1975), but hospitalization is an experience that disrupts all facets of privacy regulation, not least in the necessary establishment of temporary territory.

Crowding

Crowding is closely associated with aspects of territoriality and personal space. In this context, it should be seen as a psychological concept and separate from the physical meaning of density, which is simply a measure of people per space unit (Gifford 1987). Altman (1975) explains crowding as a personal subjective reaction and an interpersonal process. It is regarded as the consequences of unsuccessful privacy-regulating mechanisms; thus, achieved privacy is less than desired privacy, causing psychological and physiological stress.

A widely discussed unusual study was conducted by Middlemist et al (1976, cited in Meisenhelder 1982). A hidden camera in a men's lavatory measured the time interval needed for onset of urination in relation to the proximity of an adjacent occupied urinal. The results were conclusive in that urination took longer to begin and lasted less time when personal space was crowded. Whilst this is a somewhat idiosyncratic study, it is highly relevant to nursing, since normally private occasions are routinely encroached upon.

APPLICATION TO NURSING

Returning for a moment to the introductory 'proxemic dance', the regulatory *pas de deux* was brought to a halt because of the disabling of a person handicapped by the position of being a patient. The close proximity of the nurse is inescapable as the patient is compromised in a supine position.

The concept of personal space cannot be isolated, uprooted and imposed upon a simple situation. Related concepts interact and formulate many of the variable antecedents previously discussed. Purely to examine the significance of personal space for hospitalized individuals is to ignore the reality of their experience.

Illness is a threat to security; it is not chosen and permeates as an unwelcome intruder (Lebacqz 1985). When illness occurs, one is invaded to the core and it is more important than ever to be in the place of one's choosing, a familiar territory offering safety, privacy, autonomy and self-identity, the four functions of territoriality (Hayter 1981). However, deterioration in health status frequently demands that individuals leave their territory, at least temporarily, to be placed amidst appropriate resources. Already anxious and threatened by virtue of being ill, the loss or invasion of the person's territory only fuels that anxiety.

Institutions in and of themselves interfere with all four functions of territoriality. There may be little or no privacy; indeed, as Frank (1993) describes:

Hospitals depend upon a myth of privacy. As soon as a curtain is pulled, that space is defined as private and the patient is expected to answer all questions, no matter how intimate.

On admission patients rapidly recognize the territory considered as theirs. The bed dominates the centre of the rectangular parameters marked out by the suspended curtain rail. The easy chair, bedside locker and table are all compressed within the confines of this space. In an attempt to support a sense of personal and social integrity patients marks out their territory by the strategic positioning of personal belongings (Levine 1968, cited by Allekian 1973).

Anonymity is destroyed as their Christian name and surname adorn their bed. The consultant's name precedes theirs on the label, accentuating their loss of autonomy. They are no longer responsible for themselves, a fact they cannot forget with a green identity bracelet permanently fastened to their wrist. Social roles and expertise are abandoned and there is an inevitable threat to self-identity, underscored as clothes are discarded and nightwear donned:

... none of our clothes is entirely anonymous, they are all part of ourselves in a way, an extra skin, the skin we choose to show others and which we want to see ourselves (van den Berg 1972 p 32).

Meisenhelder (1982) professes that personal space is guarded perhaps more closely than any other possession, being the only remaining protection of identity. Yet, during illness, by virtue of being a patient a person cannot defend this most precious of territories against invasion, but paradoxically is less able to tolerate intrusion of it (Hayter 1981).

Having been apportioned and labelled, into this small territory will come a parade of intruders who seem to exhibit more of a right to be there than the patient has. Many nurses, because of their 24-hour presence on the ward, consider it to be their territory (Minckley 1968). In a strict sense, the patient becomes the trespasser on the territory of those health professionals legitimized to be within the hospital's walls (Stillman 1978). Perhaps the overt repercussions of this attitude can be linked with Stockwell's (1984) findings that patients regarded by nursing staff as inappropriate admissions were less popular.

In addition to losing so many familiar supports, the patient has to learn new rules in regard to their personal space (Meisenhelder 1982). Physicians, nurses, students, in fact anyone clothed in a uniform expects ready access to any area of the patient's body as determined necessary for treatment. Personal space boundaries are likely to shrink, even to the extent that the person's body is seen as being dominated by medicine, as Frank (1993) describes: 'In becoming a patient, being colonized as medical territory and becoming a spectator to your own drama, you lose yourself'.

Academia itself affords health professionals control and becomes invasive. The analysis of blood gas results or a chest X-ray, for instance, provides the clinician with intimate knowledge of a patient's body function which is unavailable and often incomprehensible to the owner. Such detailed information has been discovered in a manner that bypasses the normal conventions of interactions and circumnavigates the protective function of personal space.

Individuals seeking help from a health professional are forced into a position where they will have to let a stranger explore physical and psychological areas which are usually kept private, as Curtin (1986, cited in Davidson 1990) stated:

Under other circumstances intimate self-disclosure to anyone other than a loved one would be overwhelmingly intrusive. In essence, a therapeutic relationship is one in which artificial intimacy is imposed by need.

Yet, interestingly, it appears that patients do not perceive personal space intrusions as highly anxiety provoking. In an exploratory study of 76 patients in four Chicago hospitals, Allekian (1973) used a two-part questionnaire covering intrusions of personal space and territory. Her results indicated that anxiety with regard to territorial invasions appeared to be greater as the intrusions became more strongly associated with the patient's territory, for example, moving 'your' bedside stand, rather than 'the' chair. However, personal space intrusions did not seem to provoke such strong annoyance. The explanation given for this unexpected finding suggested that persons entering hospital anticipate a certain amount of physical contact and are psychologically prepared for these intrusions.

The study methodology could be criticized for patients were required to cognitively simulate the various scenarios and indicate what they perceived their response to be. If the actual activities were conducted and patients' responses objectively recorded, perhaps the results may differ. It would be most interesting for a comparative study to be conducted with people in another setting, substituting the word 'nurse' in the questionnaire with 'person', in order to clarify the hypothesis that the role of the nurse and the hospital setting does influence the legitimacy of personal space intrusions, accounting for the reduced anxiety.

A more direct observational technique was used by Minckley (1968) in her examination of the crowding of personal space in recovery room patients. She discovered evidence of 'civil inattention' (Goffman 1963) whereby patients forced to be physically close (approximately 2 ft) failed to recognize adjacent patients, turning away and closing their eyes. Such results could be compared with the equilibrium compensatory model proposed by Argyle & Dean (1965). However, these patients readily identified a nurse at a distance. Such findings seem to indicate that patients do not tolerate invasions of their personal space by other patients, but exceptions are made for nurses. This report prompts the question, does legitimate intrusion of personal space still constitute invasion?

Minckley (1968) attributes this to Goffman's (1963) description of certain types of persons as 'open' persons available for social contact at all times because of the uniform that they wear. There is a silent assumption that no excuse is needed in order for them to initiate social contact.

If nurses are perceived as these 'open' people, there is perhaps a tendency for nurses to treat patients as 'open' people too, regarding their uniform as some kind of passport to intrude upon a patient's personal space (Tungapalan 1982). Sommer & Dewar stated that:

. . . nurses and physicians appear to have no reluctance about intruding upon a patient's personal space. They tend to view his body as an object lacking any kind of aura or sanctity (p 323).

Most nursing procedures represent a direct intrusion into the personal space of patients (Roberts 1973, cited by Lane 1989), with nurses deciding how close to come to an individual and how much physical contact to use during communication with them. As such, nurses are responsible for assessing a patient's positive or negative response to intrusions and reacting accordingly. Unfortunately, nurses have been cited as being unaware of both their own and patients' non-verbal behaviour (Blondis 1977, Murphy 1984).

It was from this perspective that Lane (1989) devised her Territorial Intrusion Personal Space (TIPS) scale to determine female registered nurses' and male and female adult surgical patients' perceptions of intrusion. Although the age range of the population sampled was limited to between 20 and 34 years of age, Lane presented some fascinating discoveries that she labelled 'the double standard of touch'. On collating the results of the TIPS questionnaires it transpired that nurses anticipated that female patients would have more positive emotions and male patients would have more negative emotions to intrusions of personal space. In fact, the patient responses were just the opposite, with male patients having more positive reactions than females to nurses invading their personal space. This difference in perception has generally been attributed to the fact that generally, males have a larger personal space than females, so people frequently maintain a greater distance from them (Sommer 1959).

Lane also concluded that female nurses are more comfortable with closeness and touch with female patients than with males. This preference is addressed in Lawler's (1991) revealing work *Behind the Screens*. It is intriguing to note that despite a detailed exploration of how nurses learn to overcome their own socio-cultural background to conform to a professional subculture that permits the handling of other's bodies, personal space is not mentioned once.

Giger & Davidhizar (1990) note that the novice soon becomes aware that the comfort levels of patients are related to personal space and the intrusion necessary to perform nursing tasks contravenes social norms and contributes greatly to embarrassment. From the findings cited, however, it appears that through continuous socialization and repeated exposure, nurses become desensitized to the breaking of 'distance rules'. Several writers (Hines 1985, Tungapalan 1982, White 1991) have highlighted the need for nurses to become consciously aware and responsive to a patient's spatial requirements. As White (1991) succinctly stated: 'First of all, before poking, probing, percussing or auscultating, we should stop at the social zone and introduce ourselves'.

The observant practitioner can determine from non-verbal behaviour how patients perceive their territory and personal space and how they react to intrusions (Stillman 1978). Maagenberg (1983) hypothesized that violent attacks upon staff by long-term hospitalized elderly patients could be attributed to unauthorized invasion of personal space and territory. Following a series of interviews with patients in one particular unit, it was revealed that patients wanted to be told beforehand what a staff member planned to do and that they thought staff should ask their permission before performing a nursing task. Staff awareness of these findings through a Management of Assaultive Behaviour Program resulted in a 25% reduction in time lost due to injuries to nursing personnel.

A similar *raison d'être* can be found in Mallon-Palmer's (1980, cited by Bauer 1993) interpretation of Stockwell's (1984) *The Unpopular Patient*. Patients labelled 'bad' patients were described as being complaining, bad-tempered, uncooperative and demanding. Mallon-Palmer maintains that these patients were harassed and silently resentful about intrusions of their private personal space.

So can nurses protect an invisible intangible item like personal space? In reality, whilst personal space can be differentiated and distinguished from territory, people retain their personal space boundaries within a territory, be it a public, home or temporary territory. Nursing interventions designed to assist a patient to preserve their personal space cannot ignore this fact and strategies should be developed to incorporate both concepts.

Very few writers have provided recommendations for assisting nurses in the protection of these boundaries. Those interventions that have been suggested are based upon research in proxemics and have not been systematically explored. These limited propositions will be presented within the framework devised by Aiello (1987):

1. perceived threat of invader;
2. perceived control of subject;
3. reason and circumstances surrounding invasion.

Perceived threat of invader

Firstly, it must be clarified that the nurse is perceived as the invader, in that the patient's personal space and territory are their own, albeit temporary, and are not the domain of the nursing staff. Perceived threat of nurses is a highly individual concern and referral to the expectancy/discrepancy model (Patterson 1982) is useful when exploring this.

If a patient perceives staff to be helpful and trustworthy, Ashworth (1978, cited by Bauer 1993) maintains that anxiety associated with intrusion is diminished and that continuity of nursing personnel will presumably enhance that trust. It is the nurse's responsibility to interpret by facial expression, body language, gestures, tone of voice and visual contact whether the person is distressed by closeness or not. This subtle perception should alter the manner in which the nurse practises and thereby reduces the perceived threat to the patient.

Perceived control of the subject

Studies such as those conducted by Strube & Werner (1982) have conclusively demonstrated that perceived control is directly related to the size of fluctuating personal space boundaries.

Very simple measures can be implemented by the nurse to enhance the patient's perceived level of control. There is no reason why simple courtesies that are extended in typical everyday interactions should not be exchanged in the clinical setting. Knocking before entering a room, announcing oneself behind closed curtains and introducing oneself before launching into any intrusive procedures are all straightforward ways which allow patients to prepare for entry into their personal space. It is important for nurses to realize that even simple actions such as measuring someone's radial pulse rate require a significant intrusion into personal space. When else would you tolerate a stranger holding your wrist for 30 seconds?

Asking permission before administering care also extends to tampering with physically invasive devices, such as urinary catheters, intravenous infusions and syringe drivers. All too often nurses alter settings, empty bags and so on without perceiving that these items have been incorporated into a person's personal space and unexplained interference with these appendages is tantamount to an unsolicited intrusion. It is interesting to note that Smith (1989) goes a stage further in proposing that the critically ill patient may perceive the ventilator as an extension of self, a conceptualization that she attributes to distorted proprioception from sensory deprivation.

Meisenhelder (1982) also suggests that the nurse is responsible for providing an environment that preserves a patient's personal space. Light, noise and smell all represent sensory intrusions that have significant implications for a patient's perceived level of control.

An individual's sense of distance is based upon an upright position and Summer (1979) recommends that nurses should avoid looking down on patients and instead raise the bed to give patients a stronger perspective upon their boundaries.

Reasons and circumstances surrounding intrusion

It has already been stated that nursing by virtue of its very nature will infringe upon an individual's personal space boundaries. When personal space must be invaded it need not be conducted in a way that is demeaning to the patient's dignity (Stillman 1978). Privacy and security can be assured by utilizing compensatory mechanisms, such as providing physical barriers and reducing eye contact during intimate procedures. Ultimately, the reason for invasion and the manner in which it is conducted will determine the patient's perceived level of control and experience of discomfort. Whilst this is a highly individual affair, nurses need to be aware that the use of space is an integral part of each encounter.

The application of the concept of personal space to nursing has been presented. It is apparent that this is currently a neglected area of concern and yet is one that is critical to the experience of hospitalization. Perhaps most significantly, nursing researchers have not questioned patients or nurses themselves about the lived experience of personal space invasion. The only anecdotal evidence discovered was written by van den Berg (1972):

> ... it happens to all of us from time to time that we are occasionally addressed by a person who encroaches upon the decent amount of space between two people talking. We find the other person standing almost on our toes, his face almost in ours, so that, however much we squint, we still only see a vague and distorted picture of his nose, eyes and his busy tongue. His presence is too physical (p 85).

IDENTIFICATION OF MODEL CASE

A model case of a concept is an everyday example of the concept under investigation. The presentation of an exemplar is an important aspect of any concept analysis and Rodgers (1989) recommends that such cases should be taken from experiences in practice whenever possible.

The description of the model case should illustrate the concept identified by including at least some of the characteristic attributes. To reiterate, the defining attributes of personal space included:

- invisibility
- portability
- fluctuating boundaries.

A hospital sideroom. The functional bed is covered with uncoordinating starched linen and a series of worn holey blankets. The metallic bedhead is partially obscured by two thin pillows and overhung by a multitude of tubes, dials and cylinders. Numerous coloured tangled leads can be traced to a monitor that is precariously suspended from the wall. Fastened to the monitor is a small helium balloon gaudily coloured with the words 'Get Well Soon!' imprinted across it.

To the left of the bed is a small bedside locker. A pink towel is draped across its open door and on the locker surface an old coffee jar of discoloured water is home to some drooping flowers. The inevitable water jug is camouflaged by a jumble of well-wishing cards. Paraphernalia conceals the table top, a stained cup and saucer, a few sweet wrappers, a couple of tissues and the omnipresent denture pot.

An aged lady is seated in the easy chair, her aura fills the room, her possessions litter the 10 by 12 ft area. This room, although a temporary domain, is filled by her personal space.

Leaning upon the table, she shakily rises from her seated position and adjusts her dressing gown slightly tighter around her shoulders. She shuffles across the room and laboriously opens the closed door.

Carefully manoeuvring down the corridor she arrives at the ward day-room. There are a series of fawn plastic coloured chairs arranged side by side, reminiscent of a surgery waiting room, an analogy that is further compounded by the mound of old magazines upon a low coffee table and a wealth of health education posters on the walls.

Alone, an old gentleman is concealed by a capacious newspaper. On hearing the lady enter the room, he glances up, proffers an acknowledging smile and moves towards her. An introductory handshake demarcates the distance the interactants maintain from each other, yet this is a moment when their personal space boundaries converge. The duo sit down. They are positioned opposite to each other, the coffee table forming the distinctive barrier delineating the boundaries of each individual's personal space.

Hardly a dramatic sensational model case, the exemplar illustrates this most universal and pervasive of phenomena, personal space. Personal space is characterized by its fluctuating boundaries and portability, as evidenced in this scenario by the elderly lady moving from an area where her space filled an entire room to a situation where the parameters were reduced to a distance of 4 ft. Whilst the space itself is invisible, the boundaries are frequently identifiable by the mass of personal possessions or use of physical barriers.

The case certainly demonstrates the simplicity of the concept. Although there seem to be an infinite number of variables, the spatial behaviour exhibited by all humans regardless of their status or situation is governed by this concept of personal space.

Under the guise of helping or healing, health professionals seem to have become oblivious to the normal regulatory and protective function of personal space. Thus it is hoped that this elementary description of an aged woman's fluctuating boundaries will stimulate an awareness of this rudimentary concept.

SUMMARY AND CONCLUSIONS

It may be naive to suggest that human beings exist within transparent spheres or bubbles, but it is clearly evident that there is a 'something', albeit a 'nothing', that regulates contact between members of our species.

Originally little more than an animated descriptive label, 'personal space' has become recognized as the spatial mechanism that moderates social interactions. Originating in the domain of ethologists and ornithologists the study of personal space has largely remained the remit of social scientists. Following a flurry of experiments within behavioural psychology in the 1960s, an interest in this concept has gradually permeated through to the nursing discipline. Even so, it is only over the past two decades that a few nurse researchers (Allekian 1973, Barron 1990, Lane 1989, Minckley 1968) have concerned themselves with the concept.

The scarcity of nursing literature and abundance of environmental psychology experiments have led to confusion and inconsistencies regarding the nature of personal space. Therefore, concept analysis was adopted as a strategy to systematically examine the multiplicity of uses of the concept and as a mechanism to guide the extraction and refinement of the meaning of personal space. The analysis was conducted utilizing a specifically adapted framework based upon Rodgers' (1989) evolutionary approach.

A methodical examination of surrogate terms and defining attributes culminated in the proposition of a conceptual definition of personal space:

Personal space can be defined as the constant territorial claim of an individual to an invisible portable space surrounding their person, enclosed by a boundary that fluctuates in response to certain variables.

Of course such a definition can only be tentatively concluded, being directly related to the ability of the investigator (Walker & Avant 1988) and furthermore, being time, culture and context dependent (Rodgers 1989).

The consideration of antecedents, consequences and referents served to illustrate the complexities of superficially isolating a concept from reality, in an attempt to identify the multiple variables that interact to influence the defined phenomena of personal space.

It is perhaps understandable that personal space has been overlooked by nursing researchers. By its very nature, personal space typically operates as an unconscious dimension and it seems that even when boundaries are violated, compensatory mechanisms are instinctual. Nevertheless, nursing does and always will impinge upon patients' personal space and an awareness of this concept is the first step towards explaining heightened anxiety and seemingly unprovoked defensive behaviour. As such the paucity of nursing research studies investigating this phenomenon is of concern and consequently is restrictive in that only mere deductions can be made for practical recommendations.

In the absence of such specific guidelines, the identification of a model case aimed to epitomize the defining attributes of personal space and in so doing, demonstrate the significance of this invisible and intangible concept. Personal space is a universal phenomenon that does not simply dissolve on entering a hospital setting. There is a need for all caring persons to realize that personal space is an integral aspect of a person and is a component of all interactions.

The subject of personal space is far from exhausted and numerous questions remain unanswered: for example, how is a patient's personal space actually affected by hospitalization? Is the hypothesis that patients expect their personal space to be intruded upon substantiated? Is this proposition supported for those patients in the community? Is the existence of personal space dependent upon the functioning of all five senses? Is personal space distorted in a person with a sensory deficit, for example blindness?

Since embarking on the journey of concept analysis, many avenues have been passed by. However, it is hoped that these avenues have been clearly signposted so that they can be investigated in the future, fulfilling an exploration of personal space, truly 'the most significant nothing'.

REFERENCES

Aiello J 1987 Human spatial behaviour. In: Stokolis I, Altman I (eds) Handbook of Environmental Psychology, volume 1. John Wiley, New York

Alexander J 1993 Space invaders. Daily Mail, 14 December, 33

Allekian C 1973 Intrusions of territory and personal space: an anxiety-inducing factor for hospitalised persons – an exploratory study. Nursing Research 22(3): 236–241

Altman I 1975 The environment and social behaviour. Brooks/Cole, Monterey

Altman I, Chemers M 1989 Culture and environment. Cambridge University Press, Cambridge

Ardrey R 1966 The territorial imperative. Dell, New York

Argyle M, Dean J 1965 Eye contact, distance and affiliation. Sociometry 28: 289–304

Àttree M 1993 An analysis of the concept 'quality' as it relates to contemporary nursing care. International Journal of Nursing Studies 30(4): 355–361

Auden W H 1965 About the house. Random House, New York

Auger J 1976 Behavioural systems and nursing. Prentice-Hall, New Jersey

Barron A 1990 Privacy: The right to personal space. Nursing Times 86(27): 28–30

Bauer I 1993 Patients' privacy: an exploratory study of patients' perception of their privacy in a German acute care hospital. Unpublished PhD thesis, University of Wales College of Medicine, Cardiff

Blondis M 1977 Non-verbal communication with patients: back to the human touch. John Wiley, New York

Capella J, Greene J 1982 A discrepency-arousal explanation of mutual influence in expressive behaviour in adult and infant-adult interaction. Communication Monographs 49: 89–114

Chinn P, Kramer M 1991 Theory and nursing: a systematic approach, 3rd edn. C V Mosby, St Louis

Davidson L 1990 Privacy: a room of their own? Nursing Times 86(27): 32–33

Diers D 1991 Editorial on academic exercises. Image: Journal of Nursing Scholarship 23(2): 70

Duke M, Novicki S 1972 A new measure and social learning model for interpersonal distance. Journal of Experimental Research in Personality 6: 119–132

Edney J, Walker C, Jordan N 1976 Is there reactance in personal space? Journal of Social Psychology 100: 207–217

Evans G, Howard R 1973 Personal space. Psychological Bulletin 80(4): 334–344

Felipe N, Sommer R 1966 Invasions of personal space. Social Problems 14(2): 206–214

Frank A 1993 The body as territory. In: Styles M, Moccia P (eds) On nursing: a literary collection: an anthology. National League for Nursing, New York

Fry A, Willis F 1971 Invasion of personal space as a function of age of the invader. Psychological Review 83: 235–245

Gibson C 1991 A concept analysis of empowerment. Journal of Advanced Nursing 16(30): 354–361

Gifford R 1987 Environmental psychology: principles and practice. Allyn and Bacon, USA

Giger J, Davidhizar R 1990 Culture and space. Advancing Clinical Care 5(6): 8–11

Goffman E 1963 Behaviour in public places: notes on the social organisation of gatherings. The Free Press, New York

Haase J, Britt T, Coward D, Leidy N, Penn P 1992 Simultaneous concept analysis of spiritual perspective, hope, acceptance and self-transcendence. Image: Journal of Nursing Scholarship 24(2): 141–147

Hackworth J 1976 Relationship between spatial density and sensory overload, personal space and systolic and diastolic blood pressure. Perceptual and Motor Skills 43: 867–872

Hall E 1966 The hidden dimension. The Bodley Head, London

Hardy M 1974 Theories: components, development, evaluation. Nursing Research 23(2): 100–106

Hayter J 1981 Territoriality as a universal need. Journal of Advanced Nursing 6: 79–85

Hines P 1985 One's own place: a case study on territorial behaviour. Nursing Forum 22(1): 31–33

Ingham R 1978 Privacy and psychology. In: Young J (ed) Privacy. John Wiley, Chichester

Kemp V 1985 Concept clarification as a strategy for promoting critical thinking. Journal of Nursing Education 24(9): 328–384

Kerr J 1985 Space use, privacy and territoriality. Western Journal of Nursing Research 7(2): 199–219

Kleck R 1969 Physical stigma task orientated interactions. Human Relations 22: 53–60

Lane P 1989 Nurse–client perceptions: touch. Issues in Mental Health Nursing 10(1): 1–13

Lawler J 1991 Behind the screens: nursing, somology and the problem of the body. Churchill Livingstone, London

Lebacqz K 1985 The virtuous patient. In: Shelp E (ed) Virtue and medicine. Reidel, Holland

Little K 1965 Personal space. Journal of Experimental Social Psychology 1(3): 237–247

Lyman S, Scott M 1967 Territoriality: a neglected sociological dimension. Social Problems 15(2): 236–249

Maagenberg A 1983 The violent patient. American Journal of Nursing 83(3): 402–403

McBride G, King M, James J 1965 Social proximity effects on galvanic skin responses in adult humans. Journal of Psychology 61: 153–157

Meisenhelder J 1982 Boundaries of personal space. Image: Journal of Nursing Scholarship 14(1): 16–19

Meleis A 1991 Theoretical nursing: development and progress, 2nd edn. J B Lippincott, London

Minckley B 1968 Space and place in patient care. American Journal of Nursing 68(3): 510–516

Mikes G 1946 How to be an alien. Penguin, London

Miller J 1973 The nature of living systems. In: Hardy M (ed) Theoretical foundations of nursing. MSS Corporation, New York

Murphy E 1984 High touch techniques for managing the environment. Nursing Management 15: 79–81

Norris C 1982 Concept clarification: evolving methods in nursing. Aspen Systems, Maryland

Paterson M 1976 An arousal model of interpersonal intimacy. Psychological Review 89: 231–249

Patterson M 1982 A sequential functional model of non-verbal exchange. Psychological Review 89: 231–249

Pluckhan M 1968 Space: the silent language. Nursing Forum 11(4): 386–397

Rodgers B 1989 Concepts, analysis and the development of nursing knowledge: the evolutionary cycle. Journal of Advanced Nursing 14: 330–335

Rogers M 1970 An introduction to the theoretical basis of nursing. F A Davis, Philadelphia

Schwartz B 1968 The social psychology of privacy. American Journal of Sociology 73: 741–752

Schwartz-Barcott D, Kim H 1986 A hybrid model for concept development. In: Chinn P (ed) Nursing research: methodology, issues and instrumentation. Aspen Systems, Maryland

Scott A 1988 Human interaction and personal boundaries. Journal of Psychosocial Nursing 26(8): 23 28

Smith S 1989 Extended body image in the ventilated patient. Intensive Care Nursing 5: 31–38

Sommer R 1959 Studies in personal space. Sociometry 22: 247–360

Sommer R 1969 Personal space: the behavioural basis of design. Prentice Hall, Englewood Cliffs

Stillman M 1978 Territoriality and personal space. American Journal of Nursing 78: 1670–1672

Stockwell F 1984 The unpopular patient. Croom Helm, London

Strube M, Werner C 1982 Interpersonal distance and personal space: a conceptual and methodological note. Journal of Nonverbal Behaviour 6: 163–170

Summer A 1979 Give your patient more personal space. Nursing, September: 56

Teasdale K 1989 The concept of reassurance in nursing. Journal of Advanced Nursing 14: 444–450

Tungapalan L 1982 Proxemics and the nurse. Philippine Journal of Nursing 17(1–2): 12–17

van den Berg J 1972 The psychology of the sickbed. Humanities Press, New York

Walker L, Avant K 1988 Strategies for theory construction in nursing, 2nd edn. Appleton and Lange, Norwalk

Westin A 1967 Privacy and freedom. Atheneum, New York

White R 1991 Using proxemics in everyday communication. AARC Times 14(10): 48–50

Wilson R 1963 Thinking with concepts. Cambridge University Press, Cambridge

Wuest J 1994 A feminist approach to concept analysis. Western Journal of Nursing Research 16(5): 577–586